Too Big to Succeed:
Profiteering in American Medicine

Also by Russell J. Andrews

Intraoperative Neuroprotection

Too Big to Succeed:
Profiteering in American Medicine

Russell J. Andrews, MD, DEd

iUniverse, Inc.
Bloomington

Too Big to Succeed: Profiteering in American Medicine

iUniverse books may be ordered through booksellers or by contacting:

iUniverse
1663 Liberty Drive
Bloomington, IN 47403
www.iuniverse.com
1-800-Authors (1-800-288-4677)

ISBN: 978-1-4759-7128-6 (sc)
ISBN: 978-1-4759-7129-3 (hc)
ISBN: 978-1-4759-7130-9 (e)

Library of Congress Control Number: 2013900529

Printed in the United States of America

iUniverse rev. date: 02/15/2013

Contents

Preface

"No physician, insofar as he is a physician, considers his own good in what he prescribes, but the good of his patient; for the true physician is also a ruler having the human body as a subject, and is not a mere moneymaker."

Plato, *The Republic*, Bk 1, 342-D

Why would a person—who has had the good fortune to be reasonably successful, both professionally and financially, in his career as a neurosurgeon—undertake the task of documenting the financial excesses of medicine in present-day America? A simple answer might lie in another quote from Plato:

"The life which is unexamined is not worth living."

Plato, *Dialogues, Apology*, 38

However, a more thoughtful approach is to consider the evolution of one's life in general and career in particular—and how that evolution qualifies one to address the topic of profiteering in American medicine. I benefited from travel at an early age, initially across the United States as a child, and then living in Australia for nearly two years during high school. No doubt the greatest influence in those early years, however, were two years (age twenty to twenty-two) spent in the Palau Islands of Micronesia as a Peace Corps Volunteer. It was perhaps the ideal antidote to undergraduate years spent in an idyllic New England setting during the birth (perhaps "miscarriage" might more appropriate) of the Vietnam War.

The contrast between American culture and Palauan culture to this day—more than forty years later—continues to stimulate and educate me. The Palauan culture and language reflected a view of life much more remote from Western (Euro-American) or even Eastern culture and language than one might imagine. An isolated Pacific island group presents a somewhat unique environment: for centuries—likely several millennia—the islanders were their own world. Although they eventually became remarkable seafarers with celestial navigation expertise, island people in essence had to live and die on the same speck of land with the same handful of compatriots. One had no escape, and thus one had to develop supreme interpersonal skills to be successful. But unlike isolated tribes in New Guinea or the headwaters of the Amazon, over the past several centuries these island people were subjected to visitations and invasions by a number of outsiders—the British, the Spanish, the Germans, the Japanese, and finally the Americans. An anecdote illustrates the Palauans' philosophical view of life regarding this parade of visitors and invaders and, in turn, the transient occupation of the Palauans' islands by each of these "people from the West" (as the outsiders were called by the Palauans):

Palau was divided geographically at that time (1960s) into municipalities or villages, each with its own chief. Each village also had a celestial body as its territorial possession. For the village of Melekeok, the moon was its celestial body. I happened to visit the chief of Melekeok in July 1969, just after the Apollo 11 moon walk by Neil Armstrong and Buzz Aldrin. He calmly announced, "Now the United States needs to pay rent to Melekeok."

It was unclear just how tongue-in-cheek he was—but clearly the Palauans had a view of life that placed their various occupiers in the category of temporary (if sometimes lethal) interlopers.

I was impressed (although not as consciously at that time) by the Palauan respect for their fellow villagers. I have never felt as safe as I did in the village—Ngardmau—where I spent my first year teaching English as a second language in their elementary school. On weekends, I would spear gun fish to provide for my adopted Palauan family; they in return made sure I was always well fed and clean clothed. If I were to overindulge in alcohol with my Palauan compatriots, I had no doubt they would make sure I would never be in danger. And I likewise felt the same devotion to them. Peace Corps Volunteers were given a modest sum—I believe $1,800—on completion of a two-year tour of duty to help economically with reintegration into US society. Although that was far less than a penny per hour "reimbursement," I have often said that the two years in Palau were the best years of my life. By their basic humanity, Palauans taught me that life need not come with a price tag.

After over two years in Micronesia, I returned to the United States thirsting for a knowledge of linguistics; I was captivated by how the Palauan language differed from Western languages, and how it reflected the deep differences between the Palauan and Western cultures. Fortunately the academic resources of Cambridge, Massachusetts—Harvard and MIT—met that thirst. My mathematical bent led to a fascination with theoretical linguistics and Chomsky's transformational grammar, but cross-cultural linguistics and child language acquisition were other intellectual joys. The opportunity to participate in early evaluation programs for the Children's Television Workshop put a real-world spin on graduate school. Perhaps the two greatest foreign policy efforts of the United States in the second half of the twentieth century have been the Peace Corps and Sesame Street. Likely both programs have created more goodwill worldwide (and thus more security) for the United States than all of our arms sales and export of television sitcoms.

Linguistics led to language and the brain; the capabilities of the human body are epitomized in the nervous system. After completing a dissertation investigating aspects of language organization in the right and left hemispheres of the brain (deemed worthy of the G. Milton Shy Award of the American Academy of Neurology), I entered medical school. My plans for specialization in neurology took a slight deviation after a summer spent with neurosurgeon mentors at the University of Pennsylvania; clinical neurosurgery seemed to me to be a "real-world, hands-on" brand of neurology. The US Army financed the last two years of medical school; in return I spent a year in research on high-altitude cerebral edema (brain swelling which can be fatal) and a year as an US Army Flight Surgeon in

South Korea. Like the time in Palau, Korea provided an experience in a non-Western culture—as well as the opportunity to meet my wife (now of more than thirty-two years). Somewhat similar to the Palauans, the Koreans have experienced waves of outsiders crossing their land. Perhaps this has fostered both a resourcefulness and a receptivity to outsiders and outside ideas that have no doubt been contributing factors to the remarkable transformation of South Korea from the time of my arrival (October 1979—just weeks prior to President Park's assassination) to the present. Similar transformations occurring in pockets throughout the world give hope that one's efforts toward "improving the human condition" are being mirrored by the efforts of many others, equally committed to such lofty goals, who are working diligently everywhere (alas, with varying degrees of success).

Neurosurgery residency training at Stanford began my exposure to the myriad ways in which financial reimbursement affects medical decision-making in the United States. Not only in clinical medicine, but also in medical research: when I inquired as to who in the Biochemistry Department at Stanford I might seek out to perform collagen assays on the cerebral blood vessels of patients with brain aneurysms that I had collected (to understand better the etiology of the potentially lethal brain aneurysms), I was told the faculty members had left several years earlier to form Collagen Corporation. To commercialize collagen under the umbrella of a university was not nearly as personally rewarding (financially speaking) for those professors as setting up their own company.

As my interests in brain protection during neurosurgical operations evolved during the first decade after training, I became aware of how drug companies in particular spent vast sums of money (tens of millions of dollars for each drug, involving many drugs and several companies in all) on clinical trials hoping for a "magic bullet" drug for victims of stroke or head injury. The lust for profit of these companies far exceeded the lust for objective knowledge; those of us with some knowledge of the complexities of the pathophysiology of stroke and head injury knew these trials were doomed to fail. But the Food and Drug Administration (FDA) insisted their role was not to comment on potential efficacy of drug trials—merely to insure the trials were reasonably safe for the patients (or laboratory animals) involved. For these companies, "The Decade of the Brain" (1990–1999) might well have been renamed "The Decade in Pursuit of the Dollar."

Serendipitous events—one in the early 1990s, the second a decade later—gave me the opportunity to develop collaborations with researchers at NASA Ames Research Center in Silicon Valley. The initial project (with the Smart Systems Group) resulted in the NASA "Smart Probe"—a one millimeter diameter probe using several different sensing techniques (particularly several types of optical spectroscopy) to diagnose disorders (notably cancer) in real-time. The technology initiated by NASA has been licensed to a start-up, which hopefully can bring it to clinical use in the diagnosis of breast cancer—the goal being to diagnose and treat a woman with a cancerous breast mass in one day rather than the several weeks required now (because a biopsy must be read by a pathologist before treatment can be instituted). A fringe benefit of this project has been considerable personal exposure to the world of venture capital funding for biomedical devices.

The second NASA research project—with the Nanotechnology Group—is aimed at improving our understanding of the brain-machine interface (BMI). The BMI is the heart of neuromodulation for interventions ranging from deep brain stimulation or DBS (for movement disorders such as Parkinson's disease) to neuroprostheses (devices to allow quadriplegic persons to operate an artificial or paralyzed limb, or use a computer, solely by changing the way they think). I was frustrated by the lack of understanding of how DBS works; it was just fortunate that it has been quite successful for movement disorders, but that fortune has not transferred to success with other nervous system disorders. Increasing numbers of electrodes that utilize fifty-year-old technology are being placed in various regions in the brains of patients suffering from severe depression, intractable epilepsy, and other disabling disorders refractory to medications—with outcomes that have been uncertain at best. Nanotechniques present the opportunity to interact with the nervous system at the cellular level—to understand (at that cellular as well as the larger level of brain networks) why the nervous system "misbehaves" in disorders ranging from severe depression to refractory epilepsy to unrelenting headaches to morbid obesity, among others. For me personally, the gratification is twofold: (1) we are certain to learn a great deal about how the nervous system functions in both health and disease, and (2) unlike much of modern medicine, which has become so expensive—I like to use intraoperative magnetic resonance imaging (MRI) as an example—that it will be decades before 90% of the world benefits from those techniques, nanodevices can be available worldwide very rapidly. Like cell phones, nanodevices are technically advanced but will be inexpensive when produced in large numbers. High-quality medicine should not be the exclusive province of the "1%." The National Institutes of Health (NIH) has supported the NASA Ames Nanotechnology Group on two occasions with two major grants—the more recent one being for nearly two million dollars over five years awarded to colleagues at the Mayo Clinic for collaborative development of nanodevices for neuromodulation (i.e., minute electrodes for sensing brain electrical and chemical activity). Although this amount is paltry in comparison to the amounts spent by medical device companies to market outdated technology (technology that still brings them profits, of course), the funding of the NASA (and now NASA and Mayo Clinic) projects is an encouraging step. Perhaps readers of this book will lobby their elected officials to have the appropriate regulatory and funding agencies "persuade" the medical device companies to be a bit more patient–oriented than short-term profit–oriented in the future.

I was fortunate to serve as chair of the American Association of Neurological Surgeons International Outreach Committee from 2005–2008, which gave me the opportunity to travel to many developing countries around the world. I have continued to travel, and every trip proves to be educational for me. Not only does one learn techniques for efficient and cost-effective neurosurgery using limited resources, but the use of techniques, such as telemedicine, for the advancement of health care on a large scale are being pioneered in countries outside the United States (see chapter 17). And my neurosurgery colleagues do not limit their contributions to health care. In a country where most rural schools are lucky to have a teacher and perhaps a few textbooks, a Pakistani neurosurgeon has started an elementary school in a village outside of his home town of Peshawar that has been equipped with personal computers for the students. Events like these give one the confidence that in the most unexpected places in the world good people are making good things happen.

Such acts bring to life the words of Hippocrates:

Sometimes give your services for nothing, calling to mind a previous benefaction or present satisfaction. And if there be an opportunity of serving one who is a stranger in financial straits, give full assistance to all such. For where there is love of man, there is also love of the art.

Hippocrates, *Precepts,* Ch 6

If physicians in America fail to heed the advice of their mentors from millennia ago (and if the American populace fails to demand reform of our profit-motivated health-care system), may the advice of Kent to King Lear befall us:

Kill thy physician, and the fee bestow
Upon thy foul disease. Revoke thy doom;
Or, whilst I can vent clamor from my throat,
I'll tell thee thou dost evil.

Shakespeare, *King Lear,* Act I, Scene 1

Let us hope that the health-care emperor's new clothes are not a straitjacket befitting King Lear.

Los Gatos, California
November 2012

Acknowledgments

I have been most fortunate to have a number of friends and colleagues—physicians, medical researchers, lawyers, and an author—review early drafts of this book. The response of the physicians might be summarized as "Sad but true." The response of the nonphysicians might be summarized as near-disbelief that medicine in America could have been so hijacked by the profit motive. But all have encouraged me to continue to see the project through to completion. For that support I am most grateful. Special thanks goes to my close friend of more than fifty years, Richard Fathy, who began a veritable line edit of the text with the precision of a Supreme Court legal brief. If I were Diogenes running through the streets of Athens, that solitary "honest man" would be Richard Fathy.

Thanks to my patients over nearly thirty-five years since completing medical school. Entrusting one's nervous system to another human being is perhaps the ultimate leap of faith.

Thanks also to the editorial staff at iUniverse. Their prompt and dedicated communications have made this endeavor—publishing a book such as this being a novel experience for me—as painless as possible.

Greatest thanks go to my wife Yong Sim and my family. Neurosurgery is a seductive and demanding mistress, and my wife and children have endured countless evenings and weekends without me due to the call of patient care and my commitment to efforts such as this book. Even our lovable, 100-plus-pound chocolate lab has learned not to expect too many exercise runs together, to the detriment of the health of us both. Hopefully the potential benefit of this book to health care in America will make the family sacrifice worthwhile.

It is you, the reader, who is to be thanked as well. If you are persuaded to be proactive about improving health care in America, this book will have been well worth the effort.

Introduction

Is the Emperor of Health Care Truly Naked?

Problems arise when there is a mismatch between reality and our perception of reality. In the scientific world, there are paradigms that guide the pursuit of knowledge. Experiments are constructed based on rules (guidelines based on prior experiences) to further support or disprove those paradigms. Based on how ingrained a paradigm is ("Is it based on fact or on ideology?"), changing the paradigm can be very difficult. Examples of paradigm shifts from the scientific world include the shift from "the earth is flat" to "the earth is round" and the shift from "the earth is the center of the solar system" to "the sun is the center of the solar system." People have paid dearly for their correct but unpopular point of view (e.g., Galileo was placed under house arrest for insisting that the sun, not the earth, was the center of the solar system). Scientific paradigms may not shift easily, as documented by Thomas Kuhn in *The Structure of Scientific Revolutions*.[1]

Similar problems arise in the socioeconomic world when there is a mismatch between reality and our perception of reality. Here there is not only ideology that may hinder acceptance of the mismatch, but also one's perception of his or her own personal economic benefit. In the game of life, societal good rarely trumps personal gain (or, perhaps more accurately, one's perception of personal gain). This appears to certainly be the case in the short run. For example, the cost of gasoline in the United States has for decades been around one-half the cost in most of the rest of the developed world (Europe, Japan, South Korea, Australia, etc.); yet Americans complain bitterly about any cost increase at the pump. If a dollar per gallon tax on gasoline were enacted and the funds spent on

1

highway infrastructure and mass transit, we would at some point in the very near future gain back more than our investment in terms of more rapid commutes, improved transportation safety, etc. This is not to mention the benefits of reduced dependence on imported oil and improved effect on the environment and health. Until the situation becomes intolerable (which in transportation would mean frank gridlock in commute times or a rash of collapsed bridges because of lack of maintenance), the *status quo* is difficult to change.

The current health-care system in the United States has a significant mismatch between the reality of the health care provided to the populace as a whole and the perception of that reality—at least the perception in the minds of many people in this country. Though we spend 50% more on health care per capita than other developed countries, a multitude of measures—such as life expectancy and infant mortality—indicate that we in the United States are not getting health-care value for our money. Yet many argue, often with religious fervor, against change in our health-care system. One must have "choice" (more accurately, perceived choice rather than actual choice) not "socialized medicine" (whatever "socialized medicine" means) at all costs—even if adequate health care becomes a dream for the majority of Americans because of the phenomenal personal expense. When an industry constitutes upward of one-fifth of the nation's gross domestic product (GDP)—as health care does in the United States—the perception of short-term personal gain lies in maintaining the present system. But this is the *perception*, not necessarily the reality.

This book will hopefully persuade you that today's health-care emperor, if not truly naked, has donned deceptive attire. Perhaps like the rock star who performs clothed in meat (who may thus be answering quite literally, "Where's the beef?"), the health-care system in the United States has been dressed to seduce the populace (i.e., appeal to the consumer, not the patient, in each of us). Let us hope we do not ignore the problems in today's health-care system and thus create a Galileo-like outcome—health care under house arrest! In social policy, humanity should trump ideology.

In the concluding paragraphs of his book *Supercapitalism*, Robert Reich states the following:

The purpose of capitalism is to get great deals for consumers and investors. The purpose of democracy is to accomplish ends we cannot achieve as individuals. The border between the two is breached when companies *appear* to take on social responsibilities or when they utilize politics to advance or maintain their competitive standing.[2]

The second paragraph of the Declaration of Independence begins:

"We hold these truths to be self-evident, that all men are created equal, that they are endowed by their Creator with certain unalienable Rights, that among these are Life, Liberty, and the pursuit of Happiness."

It is no mistake that the first unalienable right is the right to life. And no doubt the signatories of the Declaration of Independence had more in mind by *life* than prohibiting either abortion or the use of embryonic stem cells. They certainly had in mind the prohibition of one citizen, corporation, or the government from ending the life of another citizen. To deny citizens access to appropriate health care because profits are more important than the citizen's right to life is to violate the intent of the Declaration of Independence.

The purpose of this book is to put forward the evidence that health care in the United States in its present form violates that unalienable right to life. By converting medicine from a relationship between two persons (the patient and the physician) to corporate medicine, we—the citizens of the United States—have violated our own Declaration of Independence. We have created the archetypical breach between democracy and capitalism.

It is my civic duty as a citizen of the United States to present the evidence supporting this violation of the right to life as expressed in the Declaration of Independence.

It is your civic duty to review the evidence and draw your own conclusions—and then act on those conclusions.

Part I

Grooming the Doctor—So the Doctor–Patient Relationship Takes a Haircut!

Chapter 1: The Hippocratic Tradition—Symptoms versus Causes of the Health-Care Crisis

Medicine today in the United States is big business. To see how far it has deviated from its origins in the Western tradition, we do well to consider the Hippocratic Oath:

> I swear to fulfill, to the best of my ability and judgment, this covenant:
>
> I will respect the hard-won scientific gains of those physicians in whose steps I walk, and gladly share such knowledge as is mine with those who are to follow.
>
> I will apply, for the benefit of the sick, all measures [that] are required, avoiding those twin traps of overtreatment and therapeutic nihilism.
>
> I will remember that there is art to medicine as well as science, and that warmth, sympathy, and understanding may outweigh the surgeon's knife or the chemist's drug.
>
> I will not be ashamed to say "I know not," nor will I fail to call in my colleagues when the skills of another are needed for a patient's recovery.
>
> I will respect the privacy of my patients, for their problems are not disclosed to me that the world may know. Most especially must

I tread with care in matters of life and death. If it is given to me to save a life, all thanks. But it may also be within my power to take a life; this awesome responsibility must be faced with great humbleness and awareness of my own frailty. Above all, I must not play at God.

I will remember that I do not treat a fever chart, a cancerous growth, but a sick human being, whose illness may affect the person's family and economic stability. My responsibility includes these related problems, if I am to care adequately for the sick.

I will prevent disease whenever I can, for prevention is preferable to cure.

I will remember that I remain a member of society, with special obligations to all my fellow human beings, those sound of mind and body as well as the infirm.

If I do not violate this oath, may I enjoy life and art, respected while I live and remembered with affection thereafter. May I always act so as to preserve the finest traditions of my calling and may I long experience the joy of healing those who seek my help.[3]

Nowhere in the Hippocratic Oath is financing mentioned. Medicine is a unique relationship between two people, a relationship born of the need of one person for the skills of another person in order to live. More than even the teacher or the religious leader, the physician bears a responsibility that transcends pure financial gain. That responsibility to uphold the tradition expressed in the Hippocratic Oath has been lost in present-day medicine in the United States.

Health-care reform has been approached from the aspect of business reform in many recent publications. The salient points have become "Which reform will rein in burgeoning health-care costs?" and "Which reform will be politically acceptable?"

The causes of the health-care crisis in the United States have not been considered apart from blaming greedy malpractice lawyers, pharmaceutical companies, and health-care insurance companies. All of these are symptoms of the health-care "disease," not causes. The fact is, we have transformed health care in the United States into an industry whose goal is be profitable financially, and the health of the patient is not in the equation.

Health care is no longer a covenant between the medical professional and the patient. This book will present examples of the profit-centered aspects of health care in the United States—the symptoms of the health-care disease presently ravaging the United States. Until we admit to and examine the symptoms, it is difficult to understand the etiology or pathogenesis of the "disease"—and much more difficult still to devise a cure.

Chapter 2: Is the Physician the Cause or the Cure?
Section I: The Incoming Medical Student

Traditionally in medicine, the buck stopped with the physician. The family physician made the diagnosis and determined the best treatment based on interaction with the patient and family; the surgeon obtained informed consent and was "captain of the ship" in the operating room. The importance of the patient–physician relationship is underscored by the insistence of virtually all parties that health-care reform in the United States must maintain the sanctity of that relationship.

Have physicians abrogated that responsibility to put the patient's health and welfare above all? I would say yes—but to stop there would not be helpful in determining the causes of that abrogation. Where in the process of becoming a physician has the covenant been lost? Are physicians by nature now on a par with hedge-fund managers and unscrupulous Wall Street bankers? I think not, and hopefully I can persuade you that the etiology of today's "non-Hippocratic physician" is multifactorial—although the philosophy underlying that multifactorial etiology is maximizing profit.

One of the benefits of being a junior faculty member at most US medical schools is the opportunity to participate in various committees. One on which I sat was the Medical School Admissions Committee. The charge was to select those who would be offered acceptance to the incoming medical school class (typically eighty to one hundred students in most US medical schools) from a pool of applicants that might be ten or more times that number even after many applicants were eliminated on the basis of a noncompetitive score on undergraduate academic performance or the Medical College Admission Test (MCAT).

I was impressed by the seriousness with which my Admissions Committee colleagues undertook the selection process. Every year there were a few applicants who had spent several years with a Wall Street investment firm or a corporate legal office, but then—through an apparent epiphany in their mid- to late twenties—realized the inhumanity of their career choice and wished to pursue medicine rather than Mammon. These applicants were usually very intelligent and frequently presented excellent academic credentials. However, their motivation for the healing arts was suspect, and they rarely survived the Admissions Committee's insistence that each successful applicant have a commitment to the Hippocratic principle of noneconomic interest in medicine (e.g., experience in medical environments or other humanitarian efforts, such as Vista or Peace Corps). Having been on the faculty of four different medical schools over fifteen years, I am quite comfortable that the majority of physicians-in-training are entering medical school with a reasonably secure commitment to the Hippocratic Oath.

Thirty years ago, one might have chosen medicine as a career for its rewards of personal financial gain. However, a college student today whose goal is to secure a high income—and who does not have the entrepreneurial instincts of a Bill Gates, a Larry Page, or a Mark Zuckerberg—is much more likely to pursue a degree in business or in law rather than in medicine. Why spend four years in medical school (incurring a debt of up to several hundred thousand dollars) and three to eight years in residency (at little more than the minimum hourly wage), when in one to three years after college one can have an advanced business or law degree, which is a ticket to financial success for anyone with reasonable interpersonal skills and intelligence?

In short, the "genetic material" of the majority of physicians-to-be is unlikely to be a major factor in the ultimate outcome of the typical physician in the United States.

Chapter 3: Is the Physician the Cause or the Cure?
Section II: Training the Physician-to-Be

Medical schools and university hospitals are under tremendous financial pressure. Reimbursements for medical and surgical treatment are declining in the overall effort to reduce health-care costs. Many university hospitals—and their affiliated public or county hospitals—provide not only a disproportionate amount of unfunded or underfunded care for the uninsured, but they also are the leaders in resource-consuming cutting-edge medical/surgical treatments that are frequently loss-leaders financially. Generous faculty retirement plans from economically robust times in the past are another burden. Indeed, at one university medical center on the West Coast in the mid-1990s—a time when the economics of medical schools across the country were particularly difficult—a senior member of the university administration remarked:

> "If XX University Medical Center cannot get out of the red, XX University may get out of the business of medicine."

Apart from the Department of Veterans Affairs hospitals (which are not fee-for-service hospitals but frequently are an integral part of many medical school training programs), the faculty members of medical schools are generally incentivized to maximize the revenues from patient care, (i.e., those faculty members who generate more revenue for the medical center are rewarded financially by salary enhancements [bonuses]). Thus it is not surprising that surgery faculty members tend to perform the types of surgery that are most financially rewarding and not necessarily the types of surgery that are in the patient's best interest. Increasingly, obtaining tenure—not to mention retaining one's medical school appointment—depends not only on one's academic productivity but also on how proficient the faculty member is in maximizing his or her department's economic bottom line.

An example illustrates this: Several years ago I saw a woman in her eighties who suffered from lumbar stenosis—a condition that limits one's ability to walk and, if sufficiently severe, can affect the ability to control bowel and/or bladder function (see chapter 12). Her magnetic resonance imaging (MRI) scan of the lumbar spine clearly showed the focal stenosis, and it was recommended that she undergo lumbar decompression surgery. Such surgery removes the offending stenosis (the bone and ligaments that have hypertrophied with age), and usually entails only a twenty-four-hour hospital stay in a person of her age (indeed, in someone a decade or two younger, such surgery is frequently outpatient, [i.e., involving no overnight stay]). Being a cautious individual, she sought the opinion of another senior neurosurgeon on the faculty of a nearby academic medical center who made the same recommendation. She then sought a third opinion at a different academic medical center, where she saw a junior neurosurgeon who recommended not only the decompression surgery but also a *360° fusion*, which is placing titanium spinal fusion hardware both anteriorly (through an incision in the abdomen) and posteriorly (through an incision in the low back) (again, see chapter 12). This would involve two surgical procedures, although they can be performed under a single general anesthetic by turning the patient over after the first procedure to perform the second procedure. Not only would the risks from this unnecessarily extensive surgery be much higher than a simple decompression surgery, the patient's hospital stay and convalescence would be much longer. However, both the physician's payment and the revenue for the hospital generated by this 360° fusion surgery and the implanted hardware would be easily ten times or more than that of a simple decompression surgery.

My point here is not so much that decisions like these are wasteful of health-care dollars (not to mention presenting additional risk to an elderly patient), but rather that this decision is likely to influence the medical students and neurosurgery residents who are under the supervision of this faculty member. How can we expect the next generation of physicians to adhere to the Hippocratic Oath when their mentors are clearly motivated by financial incentives? Can one fault the faculty member, whose continued appointment will depend on the revenues he or she generates for the medical center?

Although only one example is offered here, the honest faculty member of any medical school can offer many such events. There have been instances where a particularly productive (economically speaking) physician/surgeon has been the darling of the hospital or medical center administration—only to be forced later to leave the medical staff for unscrupulous practices in the interests of maximizing financial gain both personally and for the hospital or medical center. Like a dictator whose loyalties are for the moment on our side, medical school faculty members who put revenue generation above best medical practice may be encouraged initially ("we need the dictator's oil") but fall out of favor when a line in the sand is overstepped ("that dictator cannot be allowed to massacre his own people"). In the medical scenario, the line in the sand that has been overstepped might be overzealous billing that has caught the eye of Medicare auditors or frequent patient-initiated lawsuits.

Furthermore, there is a recent trend to capitalize on the physician as a student (tuition-paying, of course!) not only through medical school but also later in one's career. For many years there have been master of public health (MPH) and doctor of public health (DrPH) programs for physicians interested in more in-depth knowledge of fields related to the traditional medical school education topics, such as biostatistics, epidemiology, environmental health, health-care policy/administration, and social/behavioral sciences. Not only are MPH degrees available from "bricks and mortar" universities, but also through completely online programs. For the physician desiring a background in the business aspects of medicine, one can pursue a master of business administration (MBA); if the interest is in the legal aspects of medicine, there is the doctor of law (Juris Doctor: JD) degree.

A more recent development in postgraduate education for physicians, which began through a partnership with the American College of Physician Executives (ACPE) in 1997, is the master of medical management (MMM) program. Approximately seven hundred physicians graduated from MMM programs over its first decade of existence. The ACPE offers the following definition of the MMM:

"Designed by senior physician executives and top faculty experts, the MMM focuses on the specific skills that CEOs, governing boards, and top managers look for in physician leaders responsible for meeting healthcare organizations' unique demands."[4]

An excerpt from the website of one such MMM program at a well-known university in California is informative:

The Business of Medicine: Health care ... continues to become more complex through policy changes, managed care consolidation, and the growing pressure to manage costs. These conditions have created a fundamental desire by physicians to take back control of the health care industry. The ... master of medical management (MMM) degree provides the formal business education physicians seek in order to realize their professional goals.[5]

In a brochure received in the mail from the same university regarding their MMM program, one of the "program highlights and benefits" includes twenty-five hours of American Medical Association (AMA) Category 1 continuing medical education (CME) credits. Additionally, the four weeks spent on-campus during the approximately one-year long program are described in thirty-three bullet points. One of the bullet points for on-campus session three, a week entitled "Strategic Planning for Growth and Profitability," is "Organizational Strategies for Developing Competitive Advantage." Interestingly (as in the website information presented above), neither the term "patient" nor any other term that could be construed to refer to the person receiving health care appears in any of these bullet points. However, the terms "financial" or "marketing" appear in seven of the bullet points.

An Internet survey was sent to 500 MMM graduates in 2005, with a response rate of nearly 50% (235 MMM graduates). The results, published in 2007, reveal interesting findings about the physicians who pursued the MMM degree.[4] The work settings for the MMM graduates were similar for ACPE members in some settings (approximately one-fourth of both groups being employed in either a group practice or a hospital setting), but MMM graduates were more likely to be in an academic health center (11% versus 4%) or health system (15% versus 4%). The motivation for seeking the MMM is telling: for 65% of respondents it was "to increase their managerial knowledge and skills," for 10% it was "to make themselves more attractive in the job market," but for only 7.5% it was "to have a greater opportunity to improve patient care." Furthermore, the work activities of MMM graduates involved 100% management-related activities (as opposed to clinical or patient care–related activities) for over 30% of the respondents, and more than 50% management-related activities for 60% of the respondents. Nearly one-fifth (19%) of respondents indicated the large percentage of time they spent in managerial activities was because of "a lack of interest in patient care."

Given the lack of concern for the doctor–patient relationship and patient care evidenced by both (1) the advertisement for the MMM program and (2) many of the MMM graduates surveyed, it is unlikely that the physicians who participated in the MMM program would gain entrance into medical school if they were returned to the ranks of the premedical school students. For some physicians, it appears that the altruistic motivation of the incoming medical student is transformed by the medical education system (medical school, residency, and postgraduate programs such as the MMM) into a desire for the managerial lifestyle and/or the most financially rewarding employment possible.

Until we consider the Hippocratic Oath (the doctor–patient relationship) to be the guiding principle of medical education instead of maximizing the medical school/hospital's profit, we cannot expect the next generation of physicians to be more responsible than the current generation. Moreover, should the American Medical Association (AMA–the parent body for certifying continuing medical education) be granting credit for physicians to pursue "educational" courses and degree programs that do not even consider the patient's welfare in the goals of their programs? As physicians, are we doing our patients a service by mastering the art of maximizing profit and competitive advantage rather than mastering the art of healing those who seek our help?

Chapter 4: Is the Physician the Cause or the Cure?
Section III: Seduction of Physicians into Corporate Medicine

Physicians are bombarded by pharmaceutical and medical device companies with gifts, lunches, and educational courses at resorts ("Bring your spouse and your golf clubs!"). It is to the credit of medical schools and the federal government that such freebies are more restricted now than in the past. But to the extent that these inducements still exist, they make truly objective decisions regarding the best care for the patient problematic.

Fortunately the reporting of potential conflicts of interest—honoraria for talks endorsing a particular company's product, investment in or membership on boards of medical (drug or device) corporations, etc.— is more universally required by law now than previously. But is merely announcing such conflicts on a slide at the end of a presentation or as a footnote at the bottom of a research publication sufficient? Is this different than the fine print in a multipage credit card agreement or mortgage application document? One expects a bank to be out to make a profit; most people put trust in their physician to be on their side. For many physicians, unfortunately, the conflict between what is the best treatment for the patient and what is the best treatment for the physician's short-term financial bottom line is often resolved in favor of improved personal finances for the physician.

Direct marketing to patients (consumers) of prescription drugs and medical/surgical treatments presents a difficult problem for physicians. One can explain why a specific drug or treatment may not be the best option for a given patient, but that may take considerable time in order to make the patient an educated consumer (which for the physician limits the number of patients who can be seen in a day). Moreover, if the patient has a firm mind-set as to the drug or treatment desired based on advertising that the patient has seen, the physician runs the risk of losing the patient to another physician if the request (e.g., for a Viagra prescription) is not honored. Fortunately in my field of neurosurgery, the vast majority of patients appreciate the time taken to educate them regarding the risks and benefits of various treatment options—and that time (plus successful surgical outcomes) results, from former patients, in a steady referral pattern of their family members, friends, and colleagues with neurosurgical complaints.

A patient treated successfully is the best form of "advertising" for a physician. I have never regretted referring a patient to another physician who may be in a better position to treat that patient. Similarly, I have ended up taking care of many patients with neurosurgical complaints over the years who were put off by another neurosurgeon who appeared too eager to pursue the surgical treatment option. Some surgeons are quite blunt in telling a patient that if he/she is not interested in surgery there is no reason for a follow-up appointment. Other surgeons use scare tactics like, "If you do not have surgery immediately, you will become paralyzed." Another tactic that sends patients running for another opinion is to propose a clearly overblown treatment, the intent of which is to generate additional income for the surgeon and revenue for the hospital rather than to provide the patient with the best odds of functional improvement with the least risk. A good example of this is the 360° fusion (anterior and posterior hardware placed in the cervical or lumbar spine), which—although necessary in some patients with marked spinal instability due to massive trauma, extensive tumor involvement of the spine, or severe osteomyelitis—is rarely indicated in patients with degenerative disorders of the spine.

Although certainly not healthy for the short-term profitability of Madison Avenue advertising agencies, placing a limit on the marketing of health-related treatments to those treatments that do not require a physician's prescription would go a long way to reducing patient-motivated "self-treatment." There is quite a difference between marketing and education with regard to medical diagnosis and treatment—but this distinction seems to be increasingly blurred in the desire to maximize short-term profits.

Chapter 5: Is the Physician the Cause or the Cure?
Section IV: Efficacy or Profitability?

<u>Low Back Pain: Profitable Panaceas</u>

Disorders of the lumbar spine, such as low back pain, lumbar stenosis, and ruptured lumbar discs, are major sources of pain, disability, and lost work. In the days before effective surgical treatments were available (roughly up until the second half of the twentieth century), many patients suffering from low back problems were treated by an extended course of bed rest (i.e., getting out of bed only to go to the bathroom) often for several weeks or more—and often with amazingly good results. These days the option of giving the human body a chance to heal itself is frequently ignored. This is as much the fault of patients—or, more correctly, our present society in general—as it is of physicians. In our "take control" culture, healing must be active (or proactive); one cannot afford to take time to let the body heal naturally. "Nobody wants an operation, but an operation can fix anything!" This is not true, but that is not the answer the type A personality wants to hear.

Several years ago, I saw a man in his late forties who came with an MRI scan of his lumbar spine showing a minimally bulging disc at one level. His complaint was, "Until a few months ago I could run seventy miles a week without pain, and now if I run seventy miles my back is sore. I can only run fifty miles a week without pain. I want an operation on this disc so I can run seventy miles a week again without pain." I tried to inform him that the human back at age approaching fifty years is not quite as durable as it is when one is decades younger—but this was not the answer he wanted to hear. He likely eventually found someone who would grant his wish for an operation (probably a 360° fusion—he had good health insurance!), but I would give 10:1 odds that he did not get back to running seventy miles a week totally pain-free due to that operation.

An intervention that can be quite effective for many people with low back pain is a lumbar support or corset. Frequently such patients come in to the office with a support belt they either purchased off the shelf at a drugstore or borrowed from a family member or friend who had low back pain—an informal support belt that has offered some measure of pain relief. But rarely are these back supports prescribed by physicians, be they primary physicians, surgeons, or pain management specialists. For years I have wondered why formal lumbar supports (fitted to the patient by an orthotist and requiring a prescription from a physician) are so rarely used, even in patients who have obtained substantial pain relief from an informal off-the-shelf lumbar support purchased at a medical supply store or a pharmacy. It appears that the reason is, "Nobody makes any money from writing a prescription for a lumbar support." Indeed, a pain management specialist—or an orthopedic surgeon or a neurosurgeon for that matter—would lose the patient (i.e., lose the financial gain) if the pain were to resolve simply with wearing a lumbar support.

Where there is pain, there is potential profit. However, unless there is a procedure, such as a steroid injection in the lumbar spine for pain control, or an operation, such as a lumbar discectomy (or better yet, an extensive lumbar fusion!), or the potential for the patient to return to the office frequently for refills of prescription pain medications—there is no profit. The orthotist who fits the patient with a lumbar support or corset derives a modest financial gain, but the physician who writes the prescription for that device does not.

In the long run, I have found that improving the patient's functionality in the most practical and minimally invasive way possible is the best medicine. That patient may not prove to be revenue-favorable for the neurosurgeon, but word-of-mouth referrals will come for various neurosurgical problems in the future from that patient's friends, relatives, and colleagues. These word-of-mouth referrals may come possibly years later; patients do not soon forget "the good, the bad, and the ugly" of encounters with physicians (especially specialists like neurosurgeons). One's own health is quite an important matter to each of us. We may soon forget a surly post office clerk or an inattentive waiter, but we are unlikely to forget a physician who attempts to convince us to pursue a treatment plan that is clearly not motivated by the potential benefit to our health, but by the benefit to the physician's own financial bottom line.

Making Profits Flow from Water on the Brain

Another example of prioritizing profitability rather than efficacy in the delivery of health care is the treatment of a condition known as normal pressure hydrocephalus (NPH). NPH is a form of communicating hydrocephalus (water on the brain), meaning the cerebrospinal fluid freely communicates between the brain and the lumbar spine but is not absorbed into the bloodstream effectively. Although the pathophysiology is poorly understood, NPH has been shown in epidemiological studies worldwide to be a significant cause of dementia in the elderly. One study in Japan published in 2008 found 2.9% of persons aged greater than sixty-five had clinical and radiological (MRI scan) features consistent with NPH.[6] Although NPH does not appear to be as common as Alzheimer's disease as a cause of dementia, fortunately for those with NPH (unlike Alzheimer's disease) there is a relatively modest surgical procedure that is quite effective in treating NPH.

The clinical picture or presentation in NPH is relatively well characterized, the classic triad being progressive dementia and memory impairment, instability of gait, and incontinence of bladder and/or bowel function. The typical appearance of the brain on the MRI scan of patients with NPH is also being increasingly refined. If the clinical picture and the MRI findings are suggestive of NPH, a relatively simple outpatient evaluation can predict which patients are likely to benefit from treatment; the evaluation consists of testing the patient's cognitive function and gait (stability and speed of walking) before and after withdrawing forty milliliters or so of cerebrospinal fluid from the lumbar spinal canal. Despite the image of a spinal tap or lumbar puncture conjured up in many people's minds, a physician experienced in performing lumbar spinal fluid withdrawal can make it a brief procedure under a local anesthetic with minimal discomfort for the patient.

The diagnosis—and treatment, if indicated—of NPH is rarely accomplished, despite the improvement in quality of life and the reduction in potentially devastating falls or other injuries from gait imbalance and memory impairment that can result from untreated NPH. In many instances, treatment could mean an elderly family member may be able to remain at home rather than be placed in a nursing home (with the nursing home's high price both financially for the health-care system as well as socially for the patient). Why is the diagnosis and treatment of this condition being neglected? Again, the economic incentives are not favorable for the physician. As the quarterly publication of the American Association of Neurological Surgeons, *AANS Neurosurgeon*, stated in an article in 2010:

> "While the direct economic benefits of placing a shunt for NPH may be limited, the indirect advantages of referring physician appreciation and family loyalty may be dramatic."[7]

In this quote, "direct economic benefits" is a euphemistic term for enhanced income for the neurosurgeon. Another publication, in 2006, used a decision analysis model to determine that many more shunts should be placed for NPH in order to maximize the benefit to society as a whole from improved quality of life of patients with NPH:

> Even if 50% of patients receiving a shunt have complications, the shunt response rate would need to be less than 5% for empirical shunt insertion to do more harm than good. Authors of most studies have reported far better statistics ... In summary, many more patients with suspected NPH should be considered for shunt insertion.[8]

Perhaps the essence of why NPH is not more frequently treated is provided by the following incident. A neuroradiology colleague, who has an interest in the use of MRI scans to help determine patients who are likely to have NPH (and who has occasionally performed an MRI scan for free on a patient with suspected NPH), recently volunteered this interchange he had with a neurologist. A patient had undergone an MRI scan that was highly suggestive of NPH. The patient's clinical picture was very consistent with NPH as well. The neuroradiologist asked the neurologist when the patient would undergo a lumbar puncture for further confirmation of the diagnosis of NPH. The neurologist's reply was, "I get forty-three dollars for doing a lumbar puncture. I can't afford to do a lumbar puncture for that reimbursement." No doubt that patient remains one who quite likely would benefit from treatment with a shunt—and would thus save society (1) the cost of hospitalizations for a fall resulting in a fractured hip or a head injury or for infections from chronic incontinence of bladder or bowel, (2) the cost of nursing home placement because the family could no longer care for the patient at home, and (3) the nonmonetary cost of social isolation and impaired quality of life.

The same neuroradiologist volunteered another encounter he had regarding NPH, this time with a senior neurosurgeon on the faculty at a major academic medical center in the area. The neurosurgeon opined that, if NPH did exist at all, it was much too frequently offered as a diagnosis. This view is contradicted by hundreds of publications from medical clinicians and researchers in the Americas, Europe, and Asia since NPH was first described in the 1960s. One must wonder whether that senior academic neurosurgeon's denial of a very well-established condition was colored by the need to see only those patients who had disorders for which the neurosurgical treatment provided a financially generous reimbursement. The pressure to be financially productive for the medical center in order to maintain progress up the academic ladder can provide a powerful distortion of reality. When health-care value is measured in dollars rather than in benefit to the patient, the power of economic realities should not be underestimated.

NPH can be treated by placing a shunt from either the lumbar spinal fluid space or the lateral ventricle of the brain to the peritoneal cavity (where the intestines are located). These two alternatives are referred to as a lumboperitoneal shunt (LPS) or a ventriculoperitoneal shunt (VPS), respectively. In either case, the shunt consists of a small, very flexible plastic tube several millimeters in diameter placed under the skin to drain spinal fluid from the nervous system to the peritoneal cavity, which easily absorbs the spinal fluid as well as the peritoneal fluid secreted to allow the intestines to slosh around freely. There is debate as to whether an LPS or a VPS is optimal to treat NPH; unfortunately, the financial aspects of placing an LPS versus a VPS appear to cloud objectivity in NPH treatment. Indeed, the financial "fog" seems to obscure objectivity with regard to optimal treatment in so many areas of medicine.

The reason for the statement in *AANS Neurosurgeon* regarding lack of "direct economic benefit" (i.e., profit for the neurosurgeon) is that the Medicare reimbursement for placing a shunt (including the preoperative visit, a roughly one-hour surgical procedure, and all follow-up care for ninety days after surgery) is approximately seven hundred dollars for an LPS and less than twelve hundred dollars for a VPS.[9] It is economically not possible for a surgeon to survive on a "surgical diet" of shunt placement operations for NPH alone; hence the procedure is much less frequently performed than would be in the best interests of patient care.

But there are strong advocates of shunting to treat NPH: the companies that make highly profitable programmable valves. A valve is essential in a VPS to prevent overdrainage of cerebrospinal fluid; a valve is not necessary in an LPS in the vast majority of patients. Programmable valves can change the resistance to spinal fluid drainage (the valve pressure) by using a programmer (a handheld telemetry unit) placed on the skin over the valve to reprogram the pressure the valve provides to restrict the spinal fluid drainage. The companies marketing programmable valves for VPS will gladly fly a neurosurgeon to Scottsdale or Las Vegas for a weekend seminar on NPH and the use of programmable valves. At five thousand dollars per programmable valve, the profit margin for the medical device manufacturer is huge. For the surgeon, there is a modest financial incentive as well to place a programmable valve, since the surgeon can be reimbursed about one hundred dollars by Medicare each time the valve is interrogated (to check the valve pressure) or reprogrammed (to a different valve pressure). Reprogramming the valve is often required in order to treat the headache that may arise from too low or too high a pressure in the cerebrospinal fluid of the brain.

Although the LPS does not require a valve (programmable or otherwise) in the vast majority of cases—and is widely used in much of the world to treat communicating hydrocephalus from various causes in addition to NPH—it is rarely used in the United States despite the advantages of the LPS over the VPS:

- Cost: The LPS, being a simple soft plastic tube, costs less than a dollar to produce (although the cost to the patient, the hospital, or the health insurance company in the United States is more than one hundred dollars); the VPS, which requires a valve, costs up to one hundred times as much to produce, and a programmable valve is worth upward of five thousand dollars in cost to the patient.
- Risk of injury at surgery: The VPS has the rare but potentially fatal risk of hemorrhage in the brain caused when the shunt is passed via a small hole drilled in the skull through the brain into the ventricle.
- Risk of infection: The VPS has a much higher infection risk than the LPS, not surprising considering its much more complicated nature (with a valve) and the much longer course under the skin (from the brain to the peritoneal cavity, rather than from the lumbar spine to the peritoneal cavity).
- Risk of shunt failure: Again, the risk is much higher with the VPS than the LPS because of its more complicated nature. This is particularly true with programmable valves used frequently with VPS; a recent publication found that the failure rate of programmable valves, when tracked for five years after placement, was much higher than for nonprogrammable valves, which cost perhaps 5% as much as the programmable valves.[10]

Despite these data supporting the use of LPS rather than VPS in the treatment of NPH (as well as other forms of communicating hydrocephalus), the use of LPS in the United States is much less frequent than in most of the rest of the world. I have repeatedly asked my colleagues from some of the most renowned academic medical centers in the United States to show me the data supporting the preference for VPS over LPS. The response is usually one based on tradition or one bordering on religious fervor rather than objective evidence (which clearly supports LPS in most situations, except in infants and very young children—who are not likely to have NPH).

NPH is a good example of a medical condition that brings out both the humanitarian and the mercenary aspects of physicians. Are these humanitarian versus mercenary tendencies genetically hard-wired into physicians? I think that is unlikely. A more likely culprit is the health-care system, which constantly pressures each member of the chain of health-care delivery to game that system in order to extract one's own portion of a shrinking health-care financial "pie." Again, the patient and the patient's welfare is not really part of the equation in this system—as our neurologist so honestly stated above.

We physicians in the United States might do well to heed our more objective colleagues in other countries, whose use of LPS to treat NPH shows a concern for patient welfare rather than for immediate personal financial gain.

Chapter 6: Eroding the Patient–Physician Relationship
Section I: Financial Issues

As mentioned previously (chapter 4), a patient who enters the doctor's office with a preconceived notion regarding the treatment to be offered can present a difficult situation for the doctor. Although one can hardly expect all information available to the health-care consumer (i.e., the patient) to be the product of totally objective studies—what is referred to as "evidence-based medicine"—it is reasonable to expect mass media (television, newspapers, and magazines) to be free of medical advertising. In the past, tobacco and alcohol were freely advertised in various media; the negative health effects of these substances have resulted in curtailing such advertising. One might similarly argue that advertising in such media for prescription medications—from drugs for sexual dysfunction and contraception to drugs for elevated cholesterol and allergies—is detrimental to the nation's overall health for several reasons:

- The billions of dollars spent by pharmaceutical companies on Madison Avenue to promote prescription drug sales before the drug's patent expires and generic drug competition steps in might be better spent on research and development of truly effective "next-generation" drugs.
- The fact that a medication requires a prescription (as opposed to being an "over-the-counter" medication) indicates that an educated decision by a health-care professional is essential for the proper use of the medication. There are sound medical reasons for requiring a prescription for many medications.

- A patient who comes to the doctor with a preconceived desire for a specific drug makes an objective doctor–patient relationship difficult.

Similarly, drug companies that provide physicians with free samples of prescription drugs may erode the objectivity of the doctor–patient relationship. A more unbiased solution to providing the patient with a trial of a medication (to determine the drug's efficacy as well as side effects in a given patient) would be to make the initial prescription of any medication free to the patient. This might be a one-week supply for some drugs or a one-month supply for others and would likely exclude certain exotic, unusual, or expensive situations, such as cancer chemotherapy drugs. This would eliminate the large expense drug companies underwrite to send out legions of "drug reps" (drug sales representatives). These drug reps (usually attractive young women) travel from doctor's office to doctor's office on a regular basis (e.g., weekly or monthly) to make certain their company's free sample drugs are readily available for the doctor to use as an inducement for patients to try their company's drug over another company's drug.

Since many doctors refuse to see drug reps, the ever-inventive Madison Avenue contingent of the pharmaceutical companies have developed twenty-first-century methods to keep their message in the doctor's eyes and ears. The company Epocrates began by providing information on drug dosing and drug interactions that could be downloaded as a program onto a doctor's PDA (personal data assistant) and, more recently, as an app onto a smartphone. However, the basic service from Epocrates being free, it became necessary to develop a revenue stream. What better way than to frontload their unbiased information on drugs with drug company infomercials? The smartphone app is free, but the drug information comes only after a pitch from a pharmaceutical company of their drug that is relevant to the medical condition for which the search has been requested. These "DocAlerts" generate $3 in sales for every $1 in drug company cost to Epocrates; reportedly over three hundred thousand physicians (and a million nurses, pharmacists, and medical students) now use Epocrates smartphone apps with DocAlerts preceding the drug information sought by the user. Epocrates's revenue is now greater than $100 million per year, more than 70% of which comes from pharmaceutical companies.[11]

Perhaps "E-Mammon" would be a more appropriate name than "Epocrates." If Hippocrates's estate had a good lawyer, there might be a lawsuit ...

Another erosion of the doctor–patient relationship has been the trend to transfer payment for office visits from the health insurance company to the patient him/herself, commonly called a "co-pay." Perhaps the motivation behind the co-pay initially was to make the patient think twice before going to the doctor—the $5 or $10 paid directly to the doctor at the time of each visit was a reminder to be prudent regarding possibly "unnecessary" visits. (In my experience, such unnecessary visits are rare; although not quite like visiting the dentist, most people have better things to do than to go to a doctor's office.) In many instances now, the office visit co-pay has morphed into a significant outlay for the patient ($40 or $50 is not uncommon). The co-pay amount may be larger than the payment received by the doctor from the insurance company itself for that patient's office visit. The doctor must insist on collection of the co-pay in order to remain financially solvent, eroding the doctor–patient relationship or— more practically for many people of limited means—resulting in canceled office visits because of the sizeable co-pay.

This point also raises the issue of whether health insurance that has such large co-pays for office visits and other treatments really is "insurance." Co-pays of 30% or more for hospital costs are not uncommon, as are deductibles of several thousand dollars per year before the insurance coverage kicks in. Many people with health-care insurance have gone bankrupt trying to meet their large co-pays and deductibles. For most people, having to pay $30,000 of a $100,000 hospital bill—not an uncommon amount for a major surgical procedure or a lengthy hospitalization for a serious medical problem—would represent a major financial burden that could lead to loss of their home and/or to bankruptcy.

One can make an analogy with education. If the student was required to make a co-pay every day in order to attend class, what would this do for school attendance? The goal in the educational system is to provide the student with the knowledge to become a productive member of society; the goal in the health-care system is to keep the patient healthy. Financial impediments are unlikely to enhance the likelihood of achieving the intended goal either in education or in health care.

Chapter 7: Eroding the Patient–Physician Relationship
Section II: Continuity of Care

The physician–patient relationship is a marriage—one that is intellectually and emotionally as intimate as the biological relationship in the traditional definition of marriage. Over the past twenty years or so, concern has been raised over the physically demanding aspect of training programs in medicine and surgery; those in training might work one hundred hours or more a week, and often twenty-four hours or longer at a time without rest or time off. Tired people make mistakes, and thus increasingly restrictive limits on how long a resident may work at one time or in a week have been implemented.

<u>Continuity of Care and the Physician-in-Training</u>
In 2003 the Accreditation Council for Graduate Medical Education (ACGME) instituted a maximum workweek of eighty hours for all physicians-in-training (residents) in the United States, in response to the perceived notion that fatigue among residents working longer hours was a significant source of medical errors leading to patient morbidity and mortality. Another justification was that limiting work hours for residents would increase the time available to improve their medical/surgical knowledge and research productivity. However, a survey and data analysis of the effect of limiting resident work hours on residents in neurosurgery (published by authors from the University of Virginia, University of Rochester, and University of Pennsylvania) came to quite a different conclusion:

> In contrast to many early assumptions, our survey and analysis have shown that most [neurosurgery training] program directors

and chief residents believe that limiting work hours can actually compromise patient care through an increase in the rate of adverse events and complications ... A study of more than three thousand patients in an urban teaching hospital has supported these findings [i.e., that when different physicians take care of patients at night there are more preventable errors and lower patient satisfaction], demonstrating that increased cross coverage led to a significant rise in potentially preventable adverse events. Such events were more than twice as likely to occur in patients covered by an intern [i.e., physician in the first year of residency training after medical school] from another team or a night-float resident than matched controls in adjacent beds (26% vs. 12%, p < 0.05).[12]

The same study provided evidence that academic performance also suffered after the residency work hours restriction was instituted. Comparing scores on the written examination of the American Board of Neurological Surgery (ABNS) for junior residents in 2002 (before the restriction was implemented) and 2006 (three years after implementation) showed a 15% decrease in 2006 (p < 0.05., statistically less than once chance in twenty of this occurring randomly). A measure of resident research productivity also declined after work hours restriction: although the number of residents attending the American Association of Neurological Surgeons Annual Meeting increased nearly 10% from 2002 to 2007, the percentage of residents attending the meeting who had abstracts for either oral or poster presentations declined from 85% to 66% (p < 0.01).[12]

Additional reports have substantiated an increase in complications following the implementation of resident work-hour restrictions in 2003 for surgical procedures in various specialties, including cardiac surgery, orthopedic surgery, and neurosurgery. One recent publication offers an explanation for the increase in morbidity seen at their institution (Neurosurgery, University of Vermont):

We hypothesize that this [i.e., increased hand-offs of patient care to different physicians] is among the reasons for increased

morbidity after introduction of the work-hour restriction ...
Our complications database is maintained by the neurosurgery
residents and attending physicians, introducing potential for
reporting bias—the disfavor for the work-hour restriction within
the neurosurgical community is well documented. A national
trend of increased perioperative complications after introduction
of the work-hour restriction favors the former hypothesis rather
than the latter.[13]

The importance of continuity of care for the physician-in-training is
highlighted in an article by the chiefs of neurosurgery at the University
of Pennsylvania, Northwestern University, and Washington University.[14]
Although the lesson may be especially important in neurosurgery, the
need for the physician-in-training in all medical and surgical specialties
to be aware of subtle changes in a patient's condition that may signal
an impending crisis—a subtle change less likely to be appreciated by
a physician who is not familiar with the patient—suggests caution in
diluting the responsibility for patient care. The authors emphasize the
patient–neurosurgeon relationship upon which the neurosurgical treatment
plan depends. Neurosurgeons-in-training must learn the importance of
knowing the patient's condition and subtle changes that may occur in that
condition. Such subtle changes, likely to be missed by a cross-covering
physician or surgeon who is not intimately familiar with the patient, may
result in a significant, possibly fatal, condition evolving that could have
been avoided with closer continuity of care. It is the patient's expectation—
and the neurosurgeon's responsibility—that the primary neurosurgeon be
available as much as possible and that "hand-offs" or cross coverage be as
limited as possible. In areas of medicine beyond neurosurgery, a similar
situation appears to be present, in that increasing the number of physicians
(who will be less familiar with the patient and the patient's condition than
the primary physician) caring for a given patient during a hospitalization
not only increases the number of complications the patient is likely to
experience but also, in the long run, is more expensive for the health-care
system as a whole.

Continuity of Care—Are the Office and the Hospital Separated by a Maginot Line?

Many family doctors and internists who have an office-based practice no longer see their patients when the patient is admitted to the hospital. Why spend possibly hours seeing patients in the hospital after a busy day seeing patients in the office? Thus a new category of physician—the hospitalist—has evolved to take care of patients only while the patients are hospitalized. In my experience there is frequently little, if any, communication between the hospitalist and the patient's primary physician, particularly if the patient is admitted at night or on a weekend when the primary physician is unavailable. Research studies have also documented the impairment in continuity of care resulting from hospitalists replacing the primary care physician when the patient is hospitalized. Universal access to the patient's complete medical record (a standardized medical database accessible to all physicians) will be a significant improvement in providing the hospitalist with the necessary medical history on a patient new to the hospitalist's care, as is the case already for integrated health-care delivery systems, such as Kaiser Permanente.

If the hospitalist were in essence the patient's primary physician while in the hospital, the requisite information would only need to reside with one physician. However, the hospitalist physician is inevitably part of a group practice and only works a shift of eight or twelve hours at a time. Thus a hospitalized patient may have up to three different primary physicians in a twenty-four-hour period. A hospitalist may be caring for twenty or more patients at a time. Is it possible for one hospitalist to "sign out" to another hospitalist every eight to twelve hours? (A sign-out consists of the outgoing physician explaining to the incoming physician each patient's current condition and treatment plan in detail.) Moreover, because of the frequent change in hospitalists, patients frequently do not know who their physician is. In fact, the patient may not have one primary physician while in the hospital—their primary physician is whoever is on call (available) at the time.

Can anything approaching the doctor–patient relationship be established with a different physician every eight to twelve hours?

Certainly the nuances of patient care—subtle changes in the patient's condition that are only evident on repeated interaction and examination but that can be crucial to optimal diagnosis and treatment—are lost when medicine adopts the tactics of tag-team wrestling. I have frequently made rounds on patients who had no idea of who his or her primary physician was while in the hospital because of the frequent changing of the guard of the hospitalists.

One recent incident brought into focus how far the doctor–patient relationship can be eroded. In order to find out which doctor would be the hospitalist taking care of an elderly gentleman who was being admitted for surgery, I called the hospital operator. I was informed that the hospitalist team in question did not have a physician-on-call schedule (i.e., the operator was not informed about who the hospitalist on call was for that hospitalist group). The operator instructed me to call the office of the hospitalist team to find out which doctor I should contact. I later ran into one member of that hospitalist team (they all are very competent and personable physicians) who explained why the hospital did not have a physician-on-call schedule for their hospitalist group:

"We have two pagers, a morning pager and an evening pager. Whoever is carrying the pager in the morning—7 a.m. until 3 p.m.—is the hospitalist on call for the morning. Whoever is carrying the pager in the afternoon and evening is the hospitalist on call for the evening."

I commented to him (only partly in jest), "So the patients' hospitalist physicians are now named 'Morning Pager' and 'Evening Pager.'"

To which he replied, in effect, "Something like that."

I then commented (I believe he took it in jest, although I am not sure myself whether I was joking or not), "Now the patient's malpractice attorney can sue the Morning Pager or the Evening Pager."

The point of this anecdote is not to be critical of the hospitalist physicians; on the contrary, for the most part they seem to be as compassionate and motivated as the physicians who are primary care providers in a one-to-one relationship with patients. However, the hospitalist system—with frequent hand-offs and dilution of the doctor–patient relationship—appears to increase the distance between the doctor and the patient (both physically and empathetically). The fact that the hospitalist physician team can morph into a nameless "Morning Pager Doc" and "Evening Pager Doc" indicates the slippery slope of diluting the responsibility for a patient's care.

Patient satisfaction and continuity of care are not the only issues in question regarding the replacement of the primary physician with a hospitalist team. A *New York Times* article summarized the findings of a large observational study regarding the overall costs of hospitalist care versus primary physician care of Medicare patients when the patients are hospitalized for medical conditions.[15] The study, published in the August 2011 issue of the *Annals of Internal Medicine*, analyzed "a 5% national sample of enrollees in Medicare parts A and B with a primary care physician who were cared for by their primary care physician or a hospitalist during medical hospitalizations from 2001 to 2006."[16] This involved more than fifty-eight thousand admissions for medical conditions to 454 hospitals over the five-year period. Patients under the care of a hospitalist physician team were on average discharged about one-half day sooner than patients under the care of a primary physician, saving Medicare an average of $282 per admission. However, during the thirty days following discharge of the patient from the hospital, the hospitalists' patients were more likely than the primary care physicians' patients to be discharged to a nursing home or rehabilitation facility rather than to be discharged home, more likely to require an emergency room evaluation and/or readmission to the hospital, and less likely to see their primary physician for a posthospitalization visit. These increased posthospitalization costs to Medicare averaged $332 per patient. Thus the apparent savings of hospitalist team care during the hospitalization evaporated (i.e., a $50 deficit resulted) when patients were followed posthospitalization. This is an excellent example of cost shifting rather than cost saving, as the authors conclude:

> Our finding of $332 more Medicare spending associated with hospitalist care in the thirty days after discharge means that all of the reduction in hospital costs shifted to costs after discharge. The cost shift might be considered modest. However, if applied to the approximate 25% of Medicare admissions cared for by hospitalists, this represents more than $1.1 billion in additional Medicare costs annually.[16]

A comment from a reader presented in the *New York Times* article summarizes the view of many medical care "consumers" (i.e., patients):

> "A good primary physician is a permanent part of your life. To hospitalists, if you drop dead on the way home, they've still done their job."[15]

It would be informative to study in more detail:

(1) the incidence of medical errors and suboptimal treatment resulting from such frequent handing-off or signing out of patients from one physician to another;

(2) the incidence of improvement in patient care due to multiple primary physicians caring for a single patient each day (i.e., two heads are better than one);

(3) patient satisfaction with multiple new nonspecialist physicians when admitted to a hospital (the hospitalist model) in contrast to having his or her primary office physician following him/her when in the hospital.

Are we creating new problems (i.e., deterioration of long-term health-care delivery) by the solution proposed for easing the burden on the office-based primary physician?

The one thing of which we can be quite certain in a health-care delivery system based on the profit motive is that the field of cost shifting (as opposed to true cost saving) will become a very profitable area in which to invest. Perhaps we should sponsor a contest to see who can devise the most palatable (i.e., deceptive) term for "cost shifting" in health care!

Chapter 8: Denouement: Dr. Hippocrates Becomes Dr. Faustus

Retirement can present a difficult decision for a physician. Given the atrophy of many physicians' incomes over the past two decades (plus the recent vicissitudes of investment-based retirement plans), medicine in the United States has become a full-time job to make ends meet. One must of course maintain the lifestyle, economically speaking, of a successful physician! This leaves little time for many physicians to cultivate a passion for golf or other similar leisure-time pursuits. The appeal of receiving remuneration for activities perceived to be less stressful than direct patient care can be hard to resist.

In the military, senior officers can leave after twenty years of service and undertake a profitable position with a defense contractor company—resulting in a comfortable supplement to military retirement benefits while functioning in a somewhat similar bureaucratic environment. For politicians, once retirement is chosen (or perhaps thrust upon them by a lost election) it becomes appealing to lobby either for the cause or the company *de jour*—or, failing that option, join a prominent law firm for one's waning years. All of these options can easily rectify the years spent on a relatively meager politician's salary.

For the senior physician, such an exit strategy also exists. In the past, under the not-for-profit situation, the structure of hospitals kept the physician "caregivers" and the hospital administrators quite separate. The physicians provided care (and had their own medical staff organization for issues such as granting hospital privileges to new physicians, maintaining quality of care, etc.) and the administrators provided the infrastructure (the physical plant, the medical supplies, information technology, etc.). Ironically, today some of the most effective (from a medical care standpoint) and efficient (from a cost standpoint) health-care organizations are those that are physician-run (e.g., the Mayo Clinic). It should not be surprising that the highest quality health care—in terms of both quality-of-life measures and patient satisfaction—results from an integrated system where the delivery of health care (i.e., the physicians and other health-care providers) is not separated from the structure of health care (i.e., the hospital administration).

With the advent of for-profit hospitals (particularly for-profit hospital chains where the hospital administration is under the leadership of a company whose headquarters are most likely in another state), the seamless relationship between the hospital's medical staff and the hospital's administrative infrastructure has disappeared. Indeed, the goal of generating the greatest profit is realized when the cost of delivering health care is minimized and the reimbursement for providing health care is maximized (i.e., the ideal situation in terms of profit is to realize handsome reimbursement while providing little or no health care). The more a for-profit health-care company can realize this model—where the physicians and the populace accept minimal health care while they pay increasingly large premiums for that dwindling health care—the more successful that health-care company will be from a business standpoint.

One of the essential aspects of this for-profit model is to convince the physicians on the hospital medical staff to be content with the flow of resources, not to medical care, but to profits. What better way to accomplish this than to have a few senior physicians join the ranks of the administration to act as spokespersons for the administration's point of view? Offer a senior physician a comfortable retainer to become a spokesperson for the for-profit hospital administration, but clothe that individual as a physician acting in the best interests of the patient. Such a person is actually a "stealth cost-containment lobbyist" more than a physician, but hospital administrators prefer terms like "chief medical officer," "chief of staff," or "medical ombudsman."

One example is that of a senior physician who for his entire professional career had been on the medical staff of a respected community-based, not-for-profit hospital in California. In the early 1990s, the economic squeeze in medicine resulted in a large nationwide, for-profit hospital chain (headquartered in an eastern state) acquiring the hospital. Our senior physician colleague bemoaned the deterioration in the physician's ability to provide the best care for his or her patients once the profit rather than the patient became the hospital's *raison d'être*. It should be noted that this physician is quite conservative in his political point of view—certainly not a "bleeding heart liberal"—but that he separated his political views from his desire for the best health care for his patients. However, over a decade later, when he was in his midsixties, he became chief of staff at that hospital with, no doubt, a significant financial benefit from the hospital administration. Ironically, being quite well-to-do, he scarcely needed the income. However, the financial ties to the for-profit hospital administration changed his views quite dramatically on the ultimate goals of the hospital.

A financial relationship between a physician in a role like chief of staff and the hospital administration can severely cloud the physician's duty to provide the best care for patients. A striking example occurred at the same not-for-profit turned for-profit hospital noted in the preceding paragraph—and two chiefs of staff who followed the physician described above. Some background on the organization of hospital-based health care in California is necessary here.

In California, except for the unique situations of government health-care delivery systems (e.g., the Veterans Administration) and an integrated health-care delivery system (e.g., Kaiser Permanente), physicians are not employees of the hospital. This arrangement tends to keep the economic aspects of health-care delivery infrastructure—apart from the physician's fees, which are almost always determined by contracts between physicians or groups of physicians and the various health insurance companies—separate from the physician's relationship with the patient while the patient is hospitalized. Nurses, on the other hand, are employed by the hospital.

One of the joint responsibilities of physicians, nurses, and the hospital administration is to maintain and ideally to improve the quality of patient care. An essential part of this responsibility includes reviewing any errors that occur in delivery of care to the patient with the goal of minimizing the possibility of such an error occurring again. Although quality assurance or quality improvement is meant to be an educational effort, statistics on numbers and severity of errors in patient care are a major benchmark for ranking hospitals on overall quality of patient care. For physicians, when an untoward outcome occurs (e.g., an unexpected death or a surgical complication), the incident is typically reviewed in a monthly group meeting of members of the department concerned (e.g., the Department of Surgery). A consensus is reached on the severity of the error in care, and the physician concerned is disciplined—ranging from close monitoring of the physician's care in similar situations in the future to expulsion from the hospital's medical staff and reporting the incident to the state medical licensing board for a truly egregious incident. The latter may result in the physician losing his or her license to practice medicine in that state.

Errors incurred by nurses are typically reviewed in a nursing quality assurance program similar to that for physicians. However, given that nurses are employees of the hospital, the quality assurance process is under the control of the hospital administration. An error (e.g., giving a patient the wrong medication or the wrong dose or at the wrong time) is documented in an incident report (i.e., a brief summary of the circumstances surrounding the error). In my experience with several academic medical centers in three states and more than a dozen community hospitals (both not-for-profit and for-profit), I have usually felt comfortable that nursing errors reported through the relevant channels usually received due consideration. This hopefully resulted in less chance of a similar error occurring in the future.

At one for-profit hospital, I noticed more than the usual number of nursing errors. When I wrote an order in the patient's chart requesting that an incident report be filed regarding one specific error, I was asked not to write anything in the patient's chart about the presumed error and that incident reports at this hospital were now handled entirely online (i.e., a nurse would submit an online form documenting the incident/error).

I wanted to be certain that appropriate steps were taken to ensure that the error would not occur again. This request not to write anything in the patient's chart regarding an incident report occurred several times, which aroused my suspicion that incident reports at this hospital might disappear into "cyberspace." Since the patient's medical record is a legal document with serious consequences if it were to be altered, I got in the habit of writing an order for any incident reports. The documentation in the patient's chart would include a request that I be notified of the results of the incident report investigation. When I failed to receive a reply (on over a half-dozen such incidents over several months), I wrote a summary of each incident and submitted those summaries to the chief of staff, anticipating that I would get some response.

No reply—verbal or written—was received, despite my leaving messages with the chief of staff requesting follow-up to my written summaries of the incidents. When the next chief of staff was in place—a person whom (from professional interactions) I knew better than the previous chief of staff—I repeated the submission of the written summaries of the incidents. This physician at least informed me verbally that he would follow up on my request; but, alas, no follow-up ensued.

It has been several years since these incidents occurred, and given the lack of response from either chief of staff or any members of the hospital administration, I have decided my patients would be safer at a hospital with a more viable form of nursing quality assurance. Were these chiefs of staff not financially tied to the hospital administration—and the hospital administration's salaries (in terms of bonuses) not tied to the short-term profitability of the hospital—it is likely that such violations of quality assurance would not take place. When one's immediate financial benefit is tied to the hospital's record looking good, true patient safety is no longer paramount.

A more recent experience illustrates that the lines are being drawn in ways that do not augur well for true patient safety when physicians become financially tied to hospital administration. A general surgeon, who had given up his clinical surgical practice, became a "facilitator" between physicians and the hospital administration, this time at a not-for-profit hospital. He called me about a proposed change in the postoperative management of my patients undergoing a specific type of spine surgery.

45

The change was clearly aimed at saving money in terms of reducing the nursing staff for postoperative patients. I stated that my concern was that the patients would be adequately monitored in the early postoperative hours, and after some discussion we determined a nurse staffing situation that appeared to meet the goal of patient safety.

One of his final comments to me was quite revealing: "I am your friend." This implied that a nonphysician administrator would only be considering how to save money, but he, as a physician turned liaison for the administration, was considering me—a physician on the hospital staff—as a colleague or a friend. My concern was not collegiality, but maintaining optimal patient care. The patient does not need friends to receive excellent care; the patient needs an entire hospital team—each link of which performs its duties without failure—to have a successful outcome. To imply that a physician is still a friend once the physician becomes a member of the administration misses the point of quality assurance.

Denouement

We have seen quite an evolution in the life cycle of the physician in the United States at present. An incoming medical student usually exemplifies the Hippocratic Oath. The retiring physician (thirty to forty years later) may take on the role of an individual who strives to reduce health-care costs no matter what the ramifications for patient safety and quality of health care—with the goal of extracting a few more dollars in personal income during the waning days of a career.

Do we really want to morph Dr. Hippocrates into Dr. Faustus?

Part II

Corporate Profit and Government Policy—Partners in Profiteering

Chapter 9: Madison Avenue—the Paparazzi of Medicine

Madison Avenue advertising's profit motivation has become engrained in the delivery of medical care in the United States. Television, in particular among the mass media, has seen a remarkable increase in the number of prescription drugs that are marketed directly to the general public. Virtually any medication is fair game for direct mass marketing to the public, so long as the ad includes the magic words, "Ask your doctor if XX is right for you!" The fine-print caveats—the last section of the commercial where the announcer's rate of speech goes into overdrive delivering a list of potential side effects—should be sobering to even the most cavalier health-care consumer.

Where should one draw the line on mass media marketing (notably via television and the Internet) of prescription medications to the general public? Why stop at drugs that lower blood cholesterol levels, that raise male sexual performance, or that offer heavenly bliss for the millions of depressed citizens?

It is surprising that Madison Avenue has not capitalized on advertising for surgical procedures and implantable devices like it has on advertising for prescription drugs. Surely the medical device and surgical equipment manufacturers deserve the same access to the populace through mass media as the prescription drug companies enjoy presently. Why not advertise surgery for obesity during the dinnertime news broadcast or the latest plastic surgery procedures during daytime talk shows? Televised Monday night football could be supported not only by commercials from breweries and junk food companies, but also by commercials from surgeons, hospitals, and medical device companies. All three—surgeons, hospitals, and medical device companies—profit handsomely from surgical interventions, such as injections or implanted neurostimulators for pain; joint replacements for degenerated shoulders, hips, and knees; and artificial discs or fusion operations for neck and low back complaints. How about advertisements for implantable devices to treat intractable headaches or epilepsy or depression, such as electrodes in the brain (deep brain stimulation) or vagus nerve stimulators? Why stop at persuading patients to take the latest prescription drug (which may not be appropriate for their condition, or which may be much more expensive than the patient's current generic drug), when electrodes in the brain for the millions of chronically depressed patients in the United States is potentially a much more lucrative market?

We can only hope that television commercials for the surgical treatment of hemorrhoids (naturally with videos of the actual procedure) would be limited to airing after the dinner hour.

Finally, let's create the "Home Shopping Network: Health Care Edition," where special prices could be advertised on drugs and surgical procedures—plus, of course, the 800 number and website of the physicians and surgeons who can "make it happen" for the consumer. Why bother with minor details like having the physician obtain the history of the illness from the patient and perform a physical examination? The goal is to be profitable, so why let minor details get in the way, such as the efficacy and benefit to the patient of the drug prescribed or the surgical procedure performed?

The point of the tongue-in-cheek examples above is that when profits trump patients, there is no end to how far the paparazzi of medicine— Madison Avenue advertising in the mass media—will go in the effort to extract the last dollar out of health care. However, there is a precedent for putting patients before profits in the mass media. When the detrimental effects of smoking and excessive alcohol consumption became too well documented to ignore, a paradigm shift occurred in what was deemed acceptable mass media advertising. The costs to society of smoking and drinking became so exorbitant that even the deep-pocketed Madison Avenue advertising corporations could not outbid the general welfare—and advertisements for cigarettes and alcohol were no longer seen in mass media such as television. Let's hope that the same sanity will appear regarding the mass media marketing of regulated drugs and devices directly to consumers (patients) by those who stand to benefit financially. It might be unreasonable to expect Madison Avenue to take the Hippocratic Oath, but it is not unreasonable to demand that mass media advertising be informative rather than seductive.

Chapter 10: Of Patents, Profits, and Patient Treatment Options

The patent system for medical drugs and devices—like the patent system for novel inventions in general—is intended to provide the inventor with a period (usually up to about twenty years) to perfect the concept, develop the drug or device for clinical use, obtain clearance from the Food and Drug Administration (FDA), and recoup the development costs (as well as make a profit, hopefully) by selling the drug or device for a decade or more. However, applying this system to the development of medical drugs and devices is frequently counterproductive to optimal patient care, as the following examples will illustrate.

Generic Drugs—Degenerating Research
A corollary of the effect of patented versus generic drugs on drug company profits is the evaporation of research on generic drugs. There is a return on investment for a drug company to pursue research on new indications (i.e., new medical conditions for which a given drug may be effective) for a drug that is under patent, but not for a drug whose patent has expired and has become generic. Why should one company invest money in research on a drug that other drug companies can then sell in competition with the company funding the research? It is unclear how large a cost is involved in such writing off of drugs whose patent has expired, but it is likely substantial. An example will illustrate this:

Traumatic brain injury (TBI) and stroke are frequent causes of brain swelling and increased pressure within the cranial vault (intracranial pressure [ICP]). If the ICP is elevated, it can compromise the blood flow to brain tissue (cerebral blood flow [CBF]), which in turn aggravates the increased ICP, since brain tissue with inadequate blood flow continues to swell. This can become a vicious cycle until the ICP equals the arterial blood pressure, at which time there is no blood flow to the brain (CBF = 0) and brain death ensues. In fact, one way to determine brain death is to perform an arteriogram by injecting a contrast agent or dye into the major arteries of the brain; if no dye can enter the blood vessels (arteries) of the brain because the ICP is elevated to the level of the arterial blood pressure, the brain tissue cannot survive and the patient can be declared "brain dead."

Two generic drugs that are commonly given to reduce ICP in TBI or stroke are mannitol and furosemide (the latter is also known as Lasix, a commonly prescribed diuretic or water pill). These two drugs are frequently used together to reduce ICP and improve CBF—preserving brain tissue and improving the patient's functional outcome. A quite elegant series of laboratory experiments with a large animal (dog) model of TBI in the 1980s sought to determine the optimal manner of giving the two drugs to maximize the reduction in ICP and the improvement in CBF.[17] Should the two drugs be given simultaneously, or should one be given before the other? The results indicated that giving the mannitol before the furosemide offered the most improvement in CBF for the longest period of time. Despite the fact that increased ICP due to TBI and stroke are very significant causes of permanent brain injury, patient suffering, and cost to society, no studies confirming these findings in humans were conducted. Why should a drug company spend resources on research that would be of significant benefit to the patients and to society but of no financial benefit to that company's financial bottom line, since any drug company can produce and sell the generic drugs mannitol and furosemide?

Approximately fifteen years after the research indicated that furosemide should be given after mannitol to maximize the benefit on CBF, we conducted a pilot study on patients who had suffered TBI and who had increased ICP.[18] Since the patients were already having their ICP monitored (routine for patients with severe TBI), we could calculate the effects of various drug regimens on the ICP and the arterial blood pressure. The only expense was the time needed to gather and analyze the data. The results of the small (eight patients) pilot study were consistent with the results found fifteen years earlier in the lab: giving furosemide after mannitol resulted in a more sustained reduction in ICP (and therefore improvement in CBF) than mannitol alone. However, since a large-scale clinical trial has not been undertaken—no drug company is interested in research that is without a significant return on investment—mannitol and furosemide continue to be used on a daily basis in head injury and stroke centers throughout the country and around the world without the benefit of definitive confirmation of the findings in the laboratory animal model.

Thousands of patients throughout the world each year could benefit from such information on commonly used generic drugs, yet there is no financial incentive in our current health-care system to seek the optimal use of these routine drugs. There are no doubt many other examples of inexpensive, effective, commonly used drugs whose benefit to patients could be optimized by further controlled studies (both in the laboratory and in clinical settings), but whose lack of patent protection and a revenue stream make obtaining that information for optimal use impractical for drug companies.

Patent Protection—or Patent Perversion?
Another technique used by large pharmaceutical and medical device companies to maximize short-term profit is the acquisition of intellectual property in order to thwart competition rather than encourage the development of effective new treatments. A typical scenario is as follows:

A start-up company (a drug or medical device in the early stage of development) or its intellectual property is acquired by a large company in order to shelve the competing drug or device until it becomes profitable to develop the drug or device to the point of clinical implementation. An existing, less effective drug or device that is currently profitable and has many years left before patent expiration is more beneficial to the company's financial bottom line in the short run than a drug or device that could replace the existing treatment (with greater efficacy) but would require significant investment to complete the clinical trials necessary for FDA approval. The drug or device may be developed when the existing treatment approaches patent expiration—or it may not, depending on the company's perception of the profitability of the drug or device at that future time.

An example comes from devices for deep brain stimulation (DBS). DBS has become an effective treatment for thousands of people with movement disorders, such as advanced Parkinson's disease and dystonia—disorders for which there are no effective drugs or for which the drugs become less effective (or develop undesirable side effects) as the disease progresses. At least eighty thousand people have had DBS electrodes placed worldwide over the past fifteen years, primarily for disorders of movement (most often advanced Parkinson's disease). With the DBS device cost for a typical patient being $15,000 to $20,000, the total cost of the implanted DBS devices over this period is likely well over $1 billion. Moreover, studies are being conducted on the efficacy of DBS for patients with various neurological conditions that often do not respond adequately to medications, for example, epilepsy, mood disorders (such as severe depression and schizophrenia), and headache as well as other problems that may respond to the appropriate form of DBS (e.g., obesity and addictions). These are much larger populations of patients than the population of patients with movement disorders—potentially tens of millions of people worldwide.

Until very recently, one major medical device company (let's call it DBS INC) had the only FDA-approved DBS device, which has been marketed worldwide and is no doubt quite profitable. The electrodes are placed through a hole in the skull deep into the brain (six centimeters or more) to provide stimulation at specific sites. The electrodes themselves use technology that has changed little in the past fifty years. Ongoing laboratory studies are demonstrating that the next generation of electrodes—including ones utilizing nanotechnology to enhance the effectiveness of neuroprotheses like DBS electrodes—will almost certainly improve the efficacy of DBS quite dramatically. DBS INC gained a broad patent in 2004 on the application of nanotechniques to DBS electrodes and to electrodes for stimulation of other tissues, such as the heart (e.g., cardiac pacemaker electrodes), with little specific supporting data. A government research lab has been developing nanotechniques for DBS electrodes as well and filed a patent application for more specific uses in DBS—but unbeknownst to the government lab, their patent application was submitted after DBS INC had filed their patent application.

There is no evidence to date that DBS INC intends to incorporate nanotechniques to improve DBS for patients until the expiration of their patents on the current (antiquated) electrodes and techniques and/or the threat of a truly competitive rival device arises. Given DBS INC's deep pockets (financially speaking) and extensive support staff, a viable competitor is unlikely to arise soon. Meanwhile the government lab continues to develop the nanotechniques for neuroprosthetic electrodes, such as the electrodes necessary for DBS, now in collaboration with a major academic medical center where clinical trials will be undertaken. That collaboration between the government and academic labs has recently (June 2011) received a nearly $2 million National Institutes of Health (NIH) grant to further the development of nanotechniques to the stage of clinical use in DBS and other neuroprosthetic applications.

The academic and government labs will address the issue of patent infringement when the next generation of DBS electrodes are ready for clinical use in patients. It would be unlikely that a company stifling medical progress for its short-term financial gain would be permitted to impede the advanced technology developed jointly by nonprofit academic and government labs. Patents are intended to protect a company from undue competition in drug/device development, not to stifle innovation—as appears to be the case here. The granting of such a broad patent on very limited data makes one wonder whether the United States Patent Office has exercised due diligence in this matter—or perhaps the Patent Office may have "bent the rules" for a large corporation with deep pockets (financially, legally, and politically).

Deep Financial Pockets—Shallow Medical Ethics

Image guidance for surgical procedures has become a standard technique for neurosurgery, as well as other surgical specialties, over the past twenty years. Image-guided surgical navigation uses the same principle as the GPS

(Global Positioning System), which can track anything from a cell phone to a jumbo jetliner by triangulation from satellites. Image-guided navigation allows a neurosurgeon, for example, to see where the instruments being used to remove a tumor deep within the brain are located, with millimeter or even submillimeter accuracy. Typically, an overhead bar two to three feet in length has two or three cameras that track the surgeon's instrument in real time during surgery (using the same triangulation principle as the GPS). The surgeon can then track surgical instruments whose images are superimposed on the preoperative MRI scan of the brain using a video monitor in the operating room.

Several of the major medical equipment companies in the United States and others in Europe have developed image guidance systems for surgery, costing hundreds of thousands of dollars each, which quickly became the standard of care for hospitals with neurosurgical departments treating intracranial tumors and other brain disorders. Within a few years, similar systems became important for precision placement of spinal fusion hardware as well.

Researchers at a major university medical center developed a competing image guidance system more than a decade ago—a system with much better video display capabilities and ease of use and at much less cost. A start-up company was formed to produce the image guidance system. When the start-up company began marketing their image guidance system to hospitals, it was very successful due to the technical and financial advantages. Having sensed the threat to their stranglehold on the image-guidance market, the major medical equipment manufacturer (which just happened to be the parent company of DBS INC) promptly reduced the price of their device to match or beat that of the start-up company. Unlike the market for a laptop computer or even a car (where true competition makes profit margins slim), the profit margin on medical devices is relatively huge—and even if they are not, a large company can afford to sell their devices at a loss initially in order to drive a start-up competitor out of business. That is exactly what happened: the better device and its start-up company succumbed to the undercutting by the entrenched major medical device manufacturer. The start-up went bankrupt, with some of their intellectual property being acquired by another medical device company.

The better medical device failed to succeed because the entrenched, dominant company was able to starve the start-up financially until it died. Given the difference in size and financial resources between a huge multinational medical device company and a nascent start-up, it might be more appropriate to compare such practices to "genocide" rather than "Darwinian survival of the fittest."

The health of all of us suffers as a consequence of the profitable companies becoming more profitable at the expense of medical progress.

Chapter 11: Decade of the Brain—or Decade of the Dollar?

Another example illustrates how short-term corporate greed compromises medical innovations. The years 1990–2000 were deemed the "decade of the brain." Both TBI and stroke are major financial burdens on our society. Each year in the United States, TBI results in more than 1.7 million people receiving medical care (emergency room or hospitalization) and more than fifty thousand deaths, with an estimated total cost (direct medical costs and indirect costs in terms of lost wages, etc.) of $60 billion.[19] Approximately eight hundred thousand people suffer a stroke each year, with an estimated total cost of over $40 billion (nearly 2/3 of that being direct medical costs).[20] It was not surprising that the major drug companies put millions of research dollars during the decade of the brain into developing a "magic bullet" drug to improve the outcome of patients suffering either a TBI or a stroke.

However, the pathophysiology of TBI and stroke (the interplay of physiological processes that results in the permanent brain injury) is very complex. The neuroscientists in major research institutions who are increasing our understanding of that pathophysiology in general agree that a single drug is unlikely to be of significant benefit alone. Almost certainly a multidrug "cocktail" will be needed to significantly improve stroke and TBI outcome. However, despite the admonitions of some of the researchers that running large, very expensive (tens of millions of dollars) clinical trials of a single drug treatment would be a waste of time, several companies proceeded to conduct these fruitless trials during the decade of the brain.

The FDA insisted its role was only to insure that the trials met safety standards—not to comment on whether the trials were likely to yield meaningful results. Having patents on different drugs, the companies refused to collaborate in the trials, which might then have included "cocktails" that would have had a much greater chance of success than the single-drug trials. Not surprisingly, none of the clinical trials for either TBI or stroke conducted by several major drug companies during the decade of the brain showed significant benefit. Not only was this a waste of likely more than $100 million (possibly much more), but the drug companies involved—being motivated by profit—have become gun-shy regarding any further drug trials for either TBI or stroke since then. Given how much of our medical progress depends on the investments of major drug and medical device companies, it would be very prudent to empower the FDA to comment on the likely benefit or success from a proposed clinical trial. Indeed, our lives depend on it.

The limitations of the present "competing corporations" model in the United States (and elsewhere) have been recently noted by none other than a senior vice president at a major pharmaceutical company in the respected journal *Nature Reviews Drug Discovery*:

> It appears that different [pharmaceutical] companies may be spending time and money pursuing targets that have already been discounted by others, rather than building on established knowledge ... If scientists were able to systematically investigate an important hypothesis, and the industry more actively shared its findings, the field would undoubtedly become more productive.[21]

For-profit drug and device companies may be likened to a habitual (but not very insightful) gambler who is attracted to those slot machines with the most bells and whistles—and not to the slot machines with the best payout odds in the long run. Since the for-profit drug and device companies are the ones who profit from the drugs and devices once they reach the clinical market (not the nonprofit academic and government laboratories, which often perform the initial studies on new drugs and devices), it behooves society in general to inform (if not restrict) these gamblers to play only those slot machines with a reasonable payout!

One might say that providing expert guidance to for-profit medical drug and device companies is "a matter of life and death"!

Chapter 12: Safety, Efficacy, Profit: Devices to Benefit the Patient or the Company Bottom Line? Examples from Lumbar Spine Surgery

Lumbar spine surgery is big business. Overall spending on lumbar spine surgery for Medicare patients alone was over $1 billion in 2003.[22] It is likely twice that at present, since the volume of lumbar spine surgery roughly doubled from 1992 to 2003 and costs over the past decade have continued to increase.[23]

Problems in the lumbar spine can be divided in to three broad categories: (1) spinal instability, (2) disc disease, and (3) stenosis. It is relatively unusual for a patient to present with only one of these three problems in isolation; many, if not most, patients have varying degrees of two or three of these broad categories of lumbar spine problems. The tripartite approach to the lumbar spine—both diagnostically and surgically—has the advantage of coinciding with the types of surgical techniques and devices that have been developed for lumbar spine problems and the divisions adopted by many of the major studies evaluating the success of lumbar spine surgery.

Lumbar Stabilization—Procedure Stable, Results Unstable, Costs Exponential

Surgical stabilization of the lumbar spine consists of performing a fusion, or spinal arthrodesis (i.e., joint fusion). Two orthopedic surgeons in New York City, Albee and Hibbs, are generally attributed with performing the first lumbar spine fusion surgeries in 1911.[24] Albee used a solid piece of bone (tibia—the large bone in the lower leg) as a graft between two lumbar spine vertebrae. Interestingly, Albee's bone-grafting techniques, developed on the eve of World War I, saved many war-wounded soldiers with limb fractures from amputation. Hibbs used small pieces of bone taken from the exposed posterior aspect of the lumbar spine; these pieces were placed in the facet joints to replace the facet joint with a bony union over time. These two techniques have served as the basis for lumbar fusion or arthrodesis surgery until the present.

Stabilization of the lumbar spine until the fusion occurred was initially achieved through bed rest (with resulting lack of stress and motion on the lumbar spine) and rigid body jackets or casts, typically made of plaster at that time. In the 1930s, metallic implants were introduced, but their use did not become widespread until the 1970s. The types of spinal stabilization implants multiplied throughout the next twenty-five years, but at a reasonably sedate rate: from 1991 to 1996 the number of lumbar fusions performed in the United States rose from 39,600 to 57,400.[25]

In 1996 the FDA approved intervertebral fusion cages—cylindrical metal devices placed between two vertebral bodies after a discectomy (disc removal) surgery in order to maintain the space previously occupied by the disc. Small pieces of bone, often taken from the patient's hip (iliac crest), were used to augment the fusion. The number of lumbar fusions performed in the United States over the five years from 1996 to 2001 more than doubled, from 57,400 to 122,000.[25] In comparison, the number of hip and knee replacement surgeries for the same period (1996–2001) increased only 15%.[22] Over the following five years (2001–2006), the number of lumbar fusion surgeries rose to about 500,000.[23] In 2003, when the number of lumbar fusion surgeries was estimated to be 250,000, the cost of the hardware implanted was estimated to be $2.5 billion. The cost in 2006 is likely to have been $5 billion or more, and by now (2012) it is likely that the hardware cost for lumbar fusion surgeries is well over $10 billion per year![23,26]

Patients with Medicare insurance represent one population for which there are relatively copious data. The magnitude of the increase in lumbar fusion surgeries over the period noted above, as well as the dramatic variation in rates of lumbar fusion surgeries in different parts of the United States, among Medicare patients is impressive. The rate of lumbar fusion surgery increased from 0.3 per 1,000 Medicare enrollees in 1992 to 1.1 per 1,000 enrollees in 2003.[22] Over the same period, the cost to Medicare for lumbar fusion surgery increased from $75 million (1992) to $482 million (2003). The cost of lumbar fusion as a percentage of all back surgery increased from 14% (1992) to 47% (2003).

Even more impressive is the regional variation in rates of back surgery in different parts of the country. Data for 2002–2003 revealed that among Medicare enrollees, the United States national average of lumbar laminectomy/discectomy (i.e., without fusion) back surgery was 2.1 per 1,000 enrollees. However, the rate of this back surgery varied from 0.6 per 1,000 enrollees in the Bronx, New York, to 4.8 per 1,000 enrollees in Mason City, Iowa—an eightfold variation. The regional variation was even more dramatic for lumbar fusion surgery: among Medicare enrollees in 2002–2003, it varied from 0.2 per 1,000 enrollees in Bangor, Maine, to 4.6 per 1,000 enrollees in Idaho Falls, Idaho—a more than twentyfold variation![22]

Are the lumbar spines of people in general, and Medicare enrollees in particular, that different in various regions of the United States? Are the spine surgeons in one city or state twenty times better (or worse) surgeons than those in another city or state? Or might a more accurate explanation be that financial motivations encourage spine surgeons in certain regions to pursue a more profitable course in their delivery of care (at least to Medicare enrollees)?

The research literature on the effectiveness of lumbar fusion using implanted hardware is clouded by many industry-supported investigations in which the results are suspect due to bias on the part of the investigators (e.g., the control group may not be truly representative or appropriate, or results that are not supportive of the particular company's instrumentation may not be published). One recent review of the lumbar spinal instrumentation literature from the Mayo Clinic came to the following conclusion:

Our review suggests that there is [sic] data supporting the thesis that lumbar instrumentation improves rates of fusion. However, there is no consistent correlation between increased rates of fusion and improved patient outcomes.[27]

63

One can be sure, however, that there is a very consistent correlation between increased rates of spinal instrumentation and the profits of the spinal instrumentation manufacturers—as well as the incomes of the surgeons who implant the devices and the balance sheets of the hospitals where the instrumentation is implanted!

"Endoscopic" Tubular Lumbar Discectomy—Sleight of Hand and Slight of Value

In patients with a clearly herniated or ruptured (as opposed to merely bulging) lumbar disc, numerous studies have shown the benefit of surgical removal of the ruptured portion of the disc over nonoperative management in terms of the patient having improvement in neurological deficits, relief of pain in the distribution of the nerve root(s) involved down either (or both) leg(s), and higher rate of return to work. Weinstein and colleagues at Dartmouth have compared surgical versus nonoperative treatment of lumbar disc herniation for up to four years following surgery in research funded by the National Institutes of Health (NIH) and other government agencies (i.e., funding sources not interested in producing data supportive of either surgical or nonsurgical treatment modality). Their findings included the following:

> At four years [postoperative], patients who underwent surgery for a lumbar disc herniation achieved greater improvement than nonoperatively treated patients in all primary and secondary outcomes except work status ... Work status showed a nonsignificant benefit for surgery at four years.[28]

One of the goals of the group at Dartmouth is to compare the economic value of different medical and surgical interventions, such as comparison of the economic benefit of surgical treatment of lumbar disc herniation with the economic benefit of antihypertensive treatment (one group being sixty-year-old males with elevated diastolic blood pressure). Regarding surgical treatment of lumbar disc herniation, they concluded:

"Our comprehensive analysis suggests that surgical treatment of herniated disc represents a reasonably cost-effective health care intervention when compared with other common health care interventions."[29]

The standard surgical procedure to treat a lumbar disc herniation is a microdiscectomy, a procedure using the operating microscope (which permits magnification up to forty times, provides 3-D visualization, and affords excellent illumination from a xenon light source). A spine surgeon experienced in microsurgical techniques can perform a microdiscectomy through an incision 1 to 1.5 inches (about 2.5 to 4 cm) long—oriented vertically along the midline of the spine directly superficial to the level of the ruptured disc. The muscle is gently dissected off the bone to allow direct visualization of the spinal canal and the region of the ruptured disc.

An endoscope is an instrument used to look inside an organ in the body. Although the first endoscope was developed over two centuries ago in Germany, endoscopy did not assume a major place in medical/surgical diagnosis and treatment until the development of miniature cameras and fiber optics beginning about fifty years ago. For many procedures, the ability to make an incision much smaller than the incision necessary for a procedure done without an endoscope is a major advantage. In laparoscopy (e.g., for gallbladder surgery or appendectomy), usually more than one small incision is made to allow separate entry points for the light source/camera and the surgical instruments. One significant drawback of endoscopy compared with the operating microscope is the lack of 3-D perception. (Endoscopic visualization is 2-D. It should be noted that 3-D endoscopes are just now reaching the stage of clinical use.) Another drawback is that one is observing the surgery on a video monitor rather than directly.

Over the past twenty years in particular, the use of endoscopy in neurosurgery has been expanding dramatically. Initially, endoscopy was used primarily for procedures within the ventricles of the brain (which are filled with cerebrospinal fluid and thus well-suited for endoscopic visualization, as opposed to, for example, a brain tumor located within brain tissue). Currently, many neurosurgeons are becoming trained in endoscopic approaches to remove pituitary tumors and base of skull tumors and to clip cerebral aneurysms—in nearly all cases with a significantly smaller incision than an "open" (i.e., using an approach through a much larger hole in the skull—a craniotomy) microscope-based procedure would require.

In 1993, a randomized, prospective trial—twenty patients in each group—comparing endoscopic discectomy with microdiscectomy was performed by neurosurgeons in Berlin who were proficient in both techniques.[30] Their technique employed an endoscope 5 mm (1/5 inch) in diameter. The results in terms of recovery of neurological function, pain control, and disability (return to work) favored the group undergoing endoscopic discectomy. Several recent prospective, randomized studies have confirmed that endoscopic discectomy appears to be as effective for lumbar disc surgery as microdiscectomy.

The differences in technique between microscopic neurosurgery and endoscopic neurosurgery (not the least being 2-D rather than 3-D perception with the endoscope) dictate that the prudent surgeon will spend considerable time with an experienced endoscopic surgeon as a mentor as well as many hours practicing in the endoscopic surgery lab before attempting an endoscopic procedure in the operating room on a patient. Numerous reports on endoscopic lumbar discectomy have stressed the importance of the surgeon being well trained in endoscopic techniques. One recent study investigated the "learning curve" for their center's first thirty patients treated with endoscopic discectomy (Groups A, B, and C being the first, second, and third ten patients, respectively):

> The complication rate was 12.5% for Group A, 10% for Group B, and 0% for Group C ... attention must be paid to the steep learning curve ... [for] this complex technique ... Obtaining [endoscopic] microsurgical experience, attending workshops, and suitable patient selection can help shorten the learning curve and decrease the complications.[31]

Over a decade ago, an enterprising company decided that there would be a lucrative market in using an endoscope for lumbar disc surgery. After all, lumbar disc surgeries are performed at least an order of magnitude more frequently than surgeries for intracranial aneurysms or pituitary tumors. They reasoned that if a spine surgeon were given a weekend-long, hands-on course in endoscopic lumbar disc surgery, the surgeon would then insist that each hospital where he/she performed lumbar disc surgery would need the equipment necessary to be an "Endoscopic Lumbar Discectomy Center" (endoscope, fiber-optic light source, and full set of instruments for endoscopic spine surgery). The equipment would cost easily tens of thousands of dollars—promising a handsome return for the company, given the hundreds of hospitals around the country where lumbar disc surgeries are performed.

Having been trained in endoscopic neurosurgery, I participated in one of these demonstrations. I was impressed by the impairment in detail of the 2-D fiber-optic endoscope in comparison with the operating microscope, and the need—because of the rigid tube of the endoscope—to pass it through the muscle one-half to one inch to the side of the spine, rather than dissecting the muscle off the spine. This parting or splitting of muscle fibers with increasingly large dilators appeared to cause as much (if not more) muscle trauma than dissecting the muscle off the spine, and it appeared to result in more postoperative muscle discomfort (requiring muscle relaxant medications) than the midline incision used in the microdiscectomy technique.

Not surprisingly, with the endoscope in the hands of surgeons not formally trained in endoscopic techniques, complications frequently occurred, such as damage to the nerve root (resulting in pain, numbness, or weakness in the affected leg), or laceration of the dura (resulting in leakage of spinal fluid). The company was forced to react quickly. Large medical device and pharmaceutical companies factor in a certain level of lawsuits as the cost of doing business—but when a rash of lawsuits surface because of the "malfunction" of a particular device or drug, eyebrows are raised both at shareholders meetings and at the FDA.

In order to salvage the device—or, more accurately, the device's market for lumbar disc surgery—the company gave up on "endoscopic discectomy" and created "tubular microdiscectomy." The endoscopic tube was enlarged (threefold, from 5 or 6 mm in diameter to 18 mm) so that, with specially designed instruments (of course—no new instruments, no new profits), the operating microscope was used to perform the surgery through the tube. The only difference between the standard microdiscectomy and the tubular microdiscectomy was splitting the muscle (to admit the now larger-diameter tube) rather than dissecting the muscle off the spine. If the disc disease or stenosis required both the right and left sides of the spine to be addressed, a separate incision and second placement of the tube through the muscle on the opposite side would be necessary. With the midline microdiscectomy approach, either side can be approached through the midline incision.

The tubular discectomy system was acquired by one of the large medical device companies in the United States. Their fact sheet (intended for media professionals and investors) claims the following "significant potential benefits" with the tubular microdiscectomy system: "1. shorter hospital stays (outpatient surgery versus two to three days with open surgery); 2. smaller scars (one inch versus up to four inches); 3. quicker return to work and normal activities; 4. avoidance of general anesthetic; 5. less postoperative pain (no muscle cutting or stripping)."[32]

Let us briefly examine each of these "potential benefits" in turn:

1. Lumbar microdiscectomy in experienced hands with a healthy patient is typically an outpatient procedure. There is no reason for a difference in postoperative hospital stay for the two procedures. In the outpatient surgery center, my lumbar disc surgery patients—like those of other spine surgeons—usually go home within several hours of completing surgery.
2. The difference in length of incision should be less than a centimeter, except in the very obese patient, where the tubular microdiscectomy incision can be shorter.
3. Regarding return to work, the major risk of lumbar disc surgery is rerupture of the disc due to too-soon return to strenuous use of

the back (lifting, bending, etc.). Postsurgical pain is very rarely a limiting factor in return to full activity in the experience of myself and many others who perform lumbar microdiscectomy surgery.

4. There is no difference between microdiscectomy and tubular microdiscectomy in the need for general anesthetic, since the procedures are identical apart from the approach used. Either approach can be performed under spinal anesthesia or local anesthesia, with similar discomfort for the patient during the procedure.

5. The discomfort caused by muscle splitting by dilation is not clearly less—and very possibly is greater in many patients—than careful dissection of the muscle tissue off the spine. This is especially the case in a bilateral procedure.

Although the company carefully avoids the use of the term "endoscopic" in their patient information regarding the "tubular microdiscectomy," many patients come with questions regarding "endoscopic discectomy"—when, in fact, they have been offered "tubular microdiscectomy." There are many websites offering information on true endoscopic discectomy, but virtually all are from private practice spine institutes or independent spine surgeons. One of the few from an academic hospital states the following:

"Presently, only select patients (about 30% of patients undergoing discectomy) are candidates for endoscopic disc surgery."[33]

To cloud the issue further, an article in a major neurosurgery journal recently reported on the use of an endoscope in conjunction with the tubular device.[34] Rather than the 5 mm diameter endoscope (with minimal tissue trauma), this study used the 18 mm diameter tubular device (more than three times as large) for access—negating the advantage of the very small incision required for the endoscope in comparison with the tubular device (which requires an incision nearly as long as standard microdiscectomy). Although the authors claim their technique is comparable if not superior to microdiscectomy, their complications—in a series of 120 patients—

included dural tears in five patients (three of whom had the tubular approach converted to an open microdiscectomy surgery for closure of the dural tears) and nerve damage resulting in permanent leg weakness in one patient (which should be extremely rare in lumbar disc surgery). Indeed, the incidence of dural tear (which usually requires placement of fine sutures or a biodegradable sealant to avoid leakage of spinal fluid postoperatively) in most series of microdiscectomy surgery is one-fourth to one-half that in this study.

Fortunately a group in the Netherlands has very recently conducted a multicenter double-blind randomized controlled trial to address the cost utility of true tubular microdiscectomy versus microdiscectomy.[35] The study involved 325 patients undergoing surgery at seven Dutch hospitals, with a one-year follow-up. The average health-care costs (initial hospitalization and surgery, formal postoperative physiotherapy, medications, reoperations) were $460 greater per patient in the tubular microdiscectomy group than in the microdiscectomy group, which did not reach statistical significance. The average societal costs (primarily lost productivity) were $1,032 greater per patient in the tubular microdiscectomy group than in the microdiscectomy group, which also did not reach statistical significance. There was a trend toward more frequent reoperation in the tubular microdiscectomy group (10 of 166 patients) versus the microdiscectomy group (7 of 159 patients). The authors observe:

"The nonsignificant differences in costs and quality-adjusted life-years in favor of conventional microdiscectomy result in a low probability that tubular discectomy is more cost-effective than conventional microdiscectomy."[35]

It is sad that a major medical device company would present such misleading information for public consumption. It appears that the First Amendment right to free speech has allowed for the "snake oil salesman" techniques of the nineteenth century to flourish in the twenty-first century. But even more disturbing is that the study noted above was performed in the Netherlands and not in the United States, where the tubular microdiscectomy device was developed. With the extraordinary expenses incurred by the US health-care system in new devices and drugs (and the government footing the bill directly for many patients, e.g., Medicare), would it not make sense for a government agency (e.g., NIH) to undertake such a definitive double-blind randomized controlled trial?

One wonders if the political influence of big business in Washington, DC, is warping our health-care system from the inside out ...

Right to life versus right to profit?

The Lumbar Stenosis Buck Stops Here—"X" Marks the STOP!

Lumbar stenosis is a condition where the spinal canal in the lumbar region becomes narrowed because of degenerative changes with aging. Lumbar stenosis can also be caused by a ruptured lumbar disc (see the preceding section) or by a tumor, but these etiologies are treated separately from the treatment strategies for degenerative lumbar stenosis. An interesting observation regarding the incidence of lumbar stenosis in the future is that diabetes mellitus (another medical condition whose incidence is rapidly increasing) appears to be a risk factor for developing lumbar stenosis. This suggests that lumbar stenosis is likely to increase among the elderly—in the United States and elsewhere—as the population ages in the future. The results of a study considering eighteen hundred patients seen over an eighteen-month period in an Orthopedic Outpatient Clinic are as follows:

"The prevalence of diabetes mellitus in the three groups (spinal stenosis, osteoporotic fracture, degenerative disc disease) was 28%, 6.5%, and 21.1%, respectively, revealing a significantly higher prevalence in the spinal stenosis group compared with the others (P = .001)."[36]

Although surgery for lumbar spinal stenosis was the fastest-growing type of lumbar surgery in the United States from 1980 to 2000, since that time the rate of surgery for lumbar spinal stenosis, at least for Medicare beneficiaries, has leveled off.[23] Indeed, from 2002 to 2007 the total number of lumbar stenosis surgeries per 100,000 Medicare beneficiaries decreased slightly from 137.4 to 135.5 (i.e., roughly a 1.4% decrease). The modest decrease in both decompression lumbar surgery (where sufficient bone is removed from the posterior part of the spine to decompress the spinal canal) and simple fusion (decompression followed by a posterior fusion, or solely an anterior fusion without posterior surgery) was offset by a marked increase in the number of complex fusion surgeries (where both anterior and posterior fusions—the so-called 360° fusion—were performed). Over the five years from 2002 to 2007, the rate of complex fusion surgeries increased from 1.3 to 19.9 per 100,000 Medicare beneficiaries—a fifteenfold increase.[23]

Other findings from this study of Medicare beneficiaries are perhaps even more concerning. Life-threatening complications occurred in 2.3% of these (mostly elderly) patients undergoing simple decompression surgery, but complications were more than twice as frequent—5.6%—in patients undergoing complex fusion surgery. Readmission to the hospital within thirty days of surgery, another indicator of surgical complications, was much more frequent in patients undergoing complex fusion surgery versus simple decompression (13% versus 7.8%). Not surprisingly, the adjusted mean hospital charges for a complex fusion surgery were much higher (nearly fourfold) than the charges for a simple decompression surgery ($80,888 versus $23,724).[22]

As we saw in the section on lumbar stabilization, a lumbar spinal fusion is of questionable long-term benefit for many of the patients who undergo these procedures. Is the motivation behind the fifteenfold increase in the use of the 360° fusion technique a desire to improve the patient's outcome and quality of life? Or is it to benefit the hospitals and medical device companies that receive the nearly $60,000 in extra Medicare costs per patient—not to mention the additional surgeon's charges for a 360° fusion, which are likely to be five to ten times the charges for a simple decompression surgery for lumbar stenosis?

A spinous process is the bone of each vertebral segment that projects posteriorly; each spinous process can be felt in the middle of the back in nonobese individuals. Separation of the spinous processes between two vertebrae where there is lumbar stenosis is accomplished by bending forward (flexion of the low back). This flexion enlarges the cross-section area of the spinal canal very slightly. Since this flexion improves the symptoms of lumbar stenosis (notably pain, cramping, or weakness in the legs), most elderly people with lumbar stenosis will prefer to walk flexed—the so-called "shopping-cart phenomenon." Placing a device between the two spinous processes accomplishes a modest enlargement of the spinal canal, similar to the flexed position. In theory, such a treatment for lumbar stenosis would be desirable, since the surgical procedure would not involve exposing the spinal canal and the nerve roots within the dura at all. Although the risks of injury to the nerve roots or dura are low when surgery is performed by an experienced and circumspect spinal surgeon, a slight risk will always be present. The essential questions are, "Will the novel device and its procedure be as, or more, successful than existing procedures?" and "Will the novel device be cost-effective?"

Perhaps even more disturbing than unnecessary 360° fusion surgeries is the creation of devices that would allow a physician—and perhaps, in the future, an untrained and unlicensed individual—to perform an invasive procedure for lumbar stenosis when the physician has had no formal training in the diagnosis and treatment of disorders of the lumbar spine (including lumbar stenosis). This appears to be a major motivation behind the development of a number of interspinous devices for the treatment of lumbar stenosis, and by extrapolation, to other diagnoses such as lumbar instability. All of these devices have in common the goal of distracting (separating) the spinous processes of two adjacent lumbar vertebrae by wedging a mass between the two adjacent spinous processes.

The original interspinous device was developed in France, not for lumbar stenosis, but as a dynamic stabilization alternative to lumbar fusion (known as the first-generation Wallis device).[37] Between 1987 and 1995, 241 patients were implanted for a variety of diagnoses, with 142 patients able to be contacted regarding their status approximately fourteen years after initial surgery. Approximately 44% of the devices were placed for lumbar stenosis, 32% for primary or recurrent lumbar disc herniation, and the remaining 24% for a combination of stenosis and disc disease or other indications. Approximately 20% of the 142 patients underwent additional lumbar spine surgery during the follow-up; three-fourths of these additional surgeries were lumbar fusions.

In the late 1990s, an orthopedic spine surgeon modified the interspinous spacer concept noted above and developed what became known as the "X-STOP" interspinous device for separating the spinous processes in the lumbar spine to treat lumbar stenosis.[38] The start-up company formed in 1997 was acquired ten years later by a large company specializing in the development and marketing of devices "to restore and preserve spinal function"; this company in turn was acquired by one of the largest medical device manufacturers in the United States six months later in 2007.[39]

That company has continued to market the X-STOP device (at a cost of about $5,500 per implant) as a treatment for lumbar stenosis. The device was approved by the FDA in 2005 based on studies that compared X-STOP to conservative (nonsurgical) treatment, not on comparison to the most appropriate surgical treatment (i.e., window laminotomy lumbar decompression through a minimally invasive microsurgical approach). On their website, the company offers data to the public comparing the X-STOP procedure with the alternative of laminectomy, citing statistics that are scarcely representative of decompressive microlaminotomy.[39] Both procedures can be performed through a 4 to 5 cm incision, both can be performed under local anesthesia (although with varying degrees of discomfort for the patient), and both should have a hospital stay of twenty-four hours or less in most patients.

Of greater concern than the lack of a valid comparison group in the trials performed to receive FDA approval is the marked discrepancy between the results presented in reports authored by the developers of the X-STOP (and who were investors in the original start-up company) and/or funded by the company marketing the X-STOP device in comparison with the results presented in reports authored by disinterested third-party spine surgeons. It is curious that one of the major reports that considered 191 patients randomized either for X-STOP surgery or for nonsurgical treatment between June 2000 and July 2001, in which the results were limited to two-year follow-up, was not published until 2006 (i.e., five years after the patients were randomized and treated). This raises the question,

"What happened to the patients later, such as, four years after surgery?" In order to have a comparison surgical group, the six (of one hundred patients in the X-STOP group initially) and the twenty-two (of the ninety-one patients in the conservative group initially) who underwent laminectomy during the study period were considered. The conclusions of the authors in this report were considerably less persuasive regarding the benefit of the X-STOP for lumbar stenosis than this position printed on the marketing company's website:

> "These results show that the X-STOP provides significant clinical improvement in the symptom severity and physical function in patients with LSS [lumbar spinal stenosis] compared with conservative therapy and is comparable with traditional lumbar decompression techniques."[38]

It is interesting that a study funded by the manufacturer of the X-STOP device presents a very positive picture of the X-STOP's value in treating lumbar stenosis.[39] The study involved 131 patients at nine centers who were moderately impaired by lumbar stenosis and who were randomized either nonoperative treatment or to placement of the X-STOP device. Twenty-one of the patients who failed nonoperative treatment underwent open surgical lumbar decompression during the two-year follow-up period. However, the data on complications, clinical effectiveness, and cost reported regarding patients who underwent open surgical lumbar decompression were taken from multiple sources, including published literature and health insurance claims data. With a large variety of data sources and analysis assumptions, the study results are presented in five tables that detail the base values, the adverse events (complications), costs for the various treatment options, cost-effectiveness of the various treatment options, and a sensitivity analysis (cost per quality-adjusted life-year) for X-STOP in comparison with nonoperative and open surgical lumbar decompression (including an option of open surgery with decompression and fusion). Why such an amalgam of data sources (much of it from outside this study) and data analyses was felt necessary is unclear. However, it did allow the authors to conclude:

> "Placement of the X-STOP spacer performed in the outpatient setting compared with LAMI [open surgical lumbar decompression] was more cost-effective than treatments such as hip replacement surgery ($2004 per quality-adjusted life-year)."[40]

We will see below that these conclusions may not hold up in comparison with data from other studies whose authors did not have the same personal financial motivation to achieve a positive result for the X-STOP. The following disclosure from the study just cited is telling:

> Corporate/industry funds were received in support of this work. One or more of the author(s) has/have received or will receive benefits for personal or professional use from a commercial party related directly or indirectly to the subject of this manuscript: for example, honoraria, gifts, consultancies, royalties, stocks, stock options, and decision-making position.[40]

A publication from Germany, one of whose authors was a consultant for the large medical device company that markets the X-STOP on both sides of the Atlantic, is sobering in comparison with the above industry-funded study.[41] In a small group of patients with lumbar stenosis studied prospectively, eleven underwent X-STOP surgery and twenty-five patients underwent microsurgical decompression with a one-year follow-up. The two groups were not comparable—they differed significantly in age and many baseline measures of severity of functional impairment—but one should be impressed that three of the eleven X-STOP patients required a second surgery within one year, while none of the patients in the microsurgical decompression group required additional surgery. From the literature, the authors estimated that a patient undergoing microsurgical decompression has a 12–18% probability of requiring reoperation during a four- to five-year follow-up period; thus they conclude that the X-STOP reoperation rate of 27% at one year was excessive.

Another report from authors completely without financial ties to the X-STOP device reported similar problems regarding the excessive reoperation rate with X-STOP.[41] In forty-six patients undergoing X-STOP surgery with a mean follow-up of thirty-four months, fourteen patients (30%) had to undergo a reoperation, and only sixteen patients (36%) reached clinical success according to the authors' criteria. Since some of their patients did quite well following X-STOP surgery, the question is how to select that roughly one-third of patients who would truly benefit from the procedure (in comparison with the nearly two-thirds of patients who achieve clinical success from microsurgical decompression surgery):

We find a success rate of only about 36% [for X-STOP] … lower than most success rates published for decompressive surgery [about 60%] … the main question that needs to be discussed is what might be the role of interspinous devices like the X-STOP in the spectrum of treatments of lumbar spinal stenosis … the current data is [sic] not enough to find predictive factors and give clear recommendations about subgroups of patients who would have the best chance of success after implantation of the X-STOP.[42]

Conclusion

What are the take-home messages from this consideration of surgical interventions for lumbar instability, lumbar disc disease, and lumbar stenosis? As we have seen in chapters 10 and 11—and will see in part III also—physicians are as much to blame as medical device companies for the plethora of expensive equipment and implants, of dubious value at the outset, that go on to fail the test of time as far as cost-effective clinical success is concerned. If a device does not appear to be of clinical value in improving patient outcomes, we physicians should not be so eager to gain short-term financial benefit by participating in trials of devices almost certain to fail in the long run. The role of government agencies, both funding agencies such as the NIH and regulatory agencies such as the FDA, could be strengthened significantly: (1) in the case of the NIH, by providing financial support in the form of grants or loans to start-up companies or academic-industrial consortiums that have a truly promising surgical technique or device; (2) in the case of the FDA, by providing guidance regarding frivolous devices submitted for regulatory approval.

Until we in the US health-care system decide that long-term efficacy— and not just short-term safety—does matter in the development and clinical implementation of health-care advances, we cannot expect to see significant improvement in the value realized for money spent on medical drug and device development. The developers and the for-profit companies will always find a way to benefit financially before the device is proven to be of limited or no clinical benefit.

One might compare the present medical device industry/culture in the United States to the "crony capitalism" that led to the recent mortgage meltdown. To quote the columnist Gene Epstein in *Barron's*, who has coined the term "crapitalism" from "crony capitalism":

> Under capitalism, profits encourage risk-taking, while losses encourage prudence. Under crapitalism, a system that too often dominates Wall Street, profits are privatized and losses socialized.[43]

One might substitute the medical drug/device industry for the banker/ mortgage lender industry as a prime example of crony capitalism; the drug/device companies pick up the profits, and the government—through services provided to Medicare, Medicaid, CHIP (Children's Health Insurance Program) beneficiaries, for example—picks up the losses when the treatments fail to perform as promised.

To those who say that such patient-benefit driven (in the case of physicians) and proactive (in the case of government support and regulatory oversight) concepts and structures represent "socialized medicine," one can cite the state and national lemon laws to protect the consumer from malfunctioning cars. One might argue that the courts and malpractice lawyers provide recourse for the health-care consumer (i.e., the patient) who suffers from a nonperforming device. However, the lemon law (in

California, for example) provides the consumer the option of trading in the nonperforming new vehicle for another new car.

To my knowledge, no lumbar spine surgeon or medical device company is able to provide the patient with a new replacement for a patient's "failed back."

Chapter 13: The Law and the Reality: Profiting from Head Injuries

Every emergency room physician is very familiar with the Emergency Medical Treatment and Labor Act (EMTALA). EMTALA, part of the Consolidated Omnibus Budget Reconciliation Act of 1985 (COBRA), was passed in 1986 by Congress within the Social Security Act, and was quickly dubbed "the antidumping statute." To quote from the Department of Health and Human Services (HHS) Centers for Medicare and Medicaid Services (CMS) 2002 Clarifying Policies Statement regarding EMTALA (CMS-1063-F):

> The Committee is most concerned that medically unstable patients are not being treated appropriately. There have been reports of situations where treatment was simply not provided. In numerous other situations, patients in an unstable condition have been transferred improperly, sometimes without the consent of the receiving hospital.
>
> There is some belief that this situation has worsened since the prospective payment system for hospitals became effective. The Committee wants to provide a strong assurance that pressures for greater hospital efficiency are not to be construed as license to ignore traditional community responsibilities and loosen historic standards.[44]

The committee revising the original EMTALA regulation sought input from the public. One comment appears to raise the issue of a patient's need to know the anticipated personal cost of care for the patient's emergency

80

medical condition (especially where the patient's insurance company might require prior authorization to cover the emergency care):

> Comment: Some commenters stated that they understood the need to avoid delaying EMTALA screening or stabilization to obtain prior authorization, but suggested that, if such authorization is not obtained, patients might be left with substantial financial responsibility. The commenters noted that individuals may request information about the costs of services while awaiting a screening examination. They stated that, while it is important to avoid even the appearance of coercion of an individual to leave the emergency department, it is also important to recognize the patient's right to be informed of potential financial liability for services (including increased liability for out-of-network services) before, rather than after, the services are furnished. These commenters recommended that the regulations be revised to state that a hospital may request financial or coverage information as long as doing so does not delay screening or stabilization. The commenters also recommended that we state that there may be discussion of the limits of an individual's health insurance coverage if the individual asks about the charges for the emergency department visit.

> Response: As noted in the Special Advisory Bulletin cited earlier (64 FR 61355), current Interpretive Guidelines indicate that hospitals may continue to follow reasonable registration processes for individuals presenting with an emergency medical condition. Reasonable registration processes may include asking whether an individual is insured and, if so, what that insurance is, as long as that inquiry does not delay screening or treatment. Reasonable registration processes should not unduly discourage individuals from remaining for further evaluation. As requested by the commenter, in this final rule, we are revising proposed §489.24(d)(4) by adding a new paragraph (iv) to clarify this policy. To avoid any misunderstanding of the requirement, we have revised the

language of the interpretative guidelines to state that reasonable registration processes must not unduly discourage individuals from remaining for further evaluation.[45]

Furthermore, neither the committee formulating the 2002 Clarifying Policies Statement regarding EMTALA, nor the committee drafting the original EMTALA regulation, expected significant economic consequences from the EMTALA regulation (in either its original or updated form):

In the preamble of the May 9, 2002, proposed rule, we stated that we believed it would be difficult to quantify the impact of the proposed changes and solicited comments on how such an impact estimate could be developed. We did not receive any comments on this point. Neither the proposed EMTALA rule published on June 16, 1988, (53 FR 22513) nor the interim final rule published on June 22, 1994, (50 FR 32086) included a quantitative analysis of the economic impact of the rule. However, in the preamble to each rule, we explained that because the great majority of hospitals do not refuse to treat individuals or transfer patients inappropriately based on their perceived inability to pay, the economic impact of those rules was minimal. Since this rule is only a modification of the previous EMTALA rules, we believe that the impact of this final rule is also minimal.[46]

Is EMTALA working? One recent study suggests that a patient's insurance status does in fact play a significant role in whether that patient is transferred to another hospital—whereas, under EMTALA, transfer can occur only for a higher level of care than can be provided by the patient's initial hospital. To quote the study's objective:

"To study the relationship between insurance status and transfer, we focused on patients with mild head injury to tease apart the medical necessity for transfer from other potential drivers, such as financial factors."[47]

A brief background aside is warranted here. The designation of certain hospitals as "trauma centers" began in the late 1960s in the United States. The American College of Surgeons has established criteria for classifying trauma centers from the most comprehensive (Level I) to less comprehensive (Level III). A Level I Trauma Center has specialists in anesthesiology, emergency medicine, and surgery in-hospital and other specialists such as critical care, orthopedic surgery, and neurosurgery on call and immediately available twenty-four hours a day, as well as trauma research and training programs. A Level II Trauma Center has similar staffing but without the research and training requirements of a Level I Trauma Center. A Level III Trauma Center has a more limited range of specialists and has transfer agreements with Level I and II Trauma Centers for transfer of patients requiring a higher level of care. Some states also recognize Level IV and occasionally Level V Trauma Centers, which have even more limited trauma resources than the Level III Trauma Centers.

The study cited above compared patients who suffered mild head injury from two data banks: the American College of Surgeons National Trauma Data Bank (NTDB) from 2002–2006 and the Massachusetts General Hospital (MGH—a Level I Trauma Center) from 1993–2009. Once patients without complete information were excluded, there were 301 NTDB patients and 181 MGH patients. Here are the principal findings of the study:

1. An uninsured patient with a mild head injury was significantly *more* likely than a similar patient with private insurance to be transferred from a Level II or III Trauma Center to a Level I Trauma Center (NTDB odds ratio: 2.07, P < .01; MGH odds ratio: 5.2, P < .01).

2. An uninsured patient with a mild head injury was significantly *less* likely than a similar patient with private insurance to be accepted in transfer (e.g., from a non–trauma center hospital) by a Level II or III Trauma Center—presumably then being sent to a Level I Trauma Center (NTDB odds ratio: 0.143, P < .01).[47]

The data seem to support the study's terse conclusion: "Insurance status appears to influence transfer patterns." However, the study was conducted by a Level I Trauma Center (MGH) because of the concern that Level I Trauma Centers are being overburdened with uninsured patients who, having only mild head injury, could be cared for adequately at a Level II or III Trauma Center. This may in fact be the case, and the study's authors go to great length discussing the myriad factors that influence the decision to transfer or accept a patient.

One might well ask for a complementary study to be conducted addressing the following question: "What is the effect of insurance status on the acceptance by Level I Trauma Centers of patients suffering a severe head injury?" In twenty-five years of having been on the neurosurgery staff of several Level I Trauma Centers, as well as Level II Trauma Centers and non–trauma center hospitals, I have seen not only the problem noted by the authors of the above study but also the problem of not being able to legitimately transfer an uninsured patient to a medical facility with the necessary higher level of care.

The most egregious example in my memory comes from an emergency room physician at a small community hospital in the southern Central Valley of California who had a patient in his emergency room with an extensive subarachnoid hemorrhage (bleeding at the base of the brain) caused by a ruptured cerebral aneurysm. The emergency room physician clearly lacked the resources at that hospital to care for the patient. He had been calling virtually every major medical center in California through the night to find a hospital to accept the patient in transfer—only to be told by each medical center that "resources were not available" (sometimes "the on-call neurosurgeon is busy with another emergency patient," but usually "we have no intensive care unit beds available right now"). On behalf of a community hospital in San Jose (about two hundred miles from the patient's hospital) where I was on staff, I agreed to take the patient in transfer. The emergency room physician called back shortly thereafter to say that a hospital in Santa Barbara, which was fortunately about one-half the distance from his hospital compared with the distance to San Jose, had just accepted the patient in transfer.

Later he kindly faxed me his telephone record for that evening; he had made repeated phone calls to nearly twenty major medical facilities with the requisite higher level of care. Every one of those medical centers claimed not to have the resources available at that time to accept his uninsured patient. The statistical probability that all of these medical centers simultaneously lacked resources must be infinitesimally small. If the patient concerned were insured rather than uninsured, no doubt this emergency room physician would have heard a response from most of these medical centers that was quite different:

"Sure, we will accept the patient in transfer immediately."

The financial game gets played both ways by the medical facilities with higher and lower levels of care. One might say that EMTALA and for-profit medicine comprise an oxymoron ...

Part III

Physicians and Physicians' Organizations: Succumbing to Mammon

Chapter 14: Medical/Surgical Turf Wars

An analogy can be drawn between the turf wars that have arisen in certain aspects of health-care delivery in the United States and the drug wars between rivaling drug cartels in our neighbor to the south, Mexico. Although not as blatantly bloody, it is certainly possible that as many lives have been lost, as much quality of life squandered, and as much economic resource wasted north of the border by the financial turf wars in medicine as south of the border in the drug cartels clashes. Three examples are given here:

Treatment of Brain Aneurysms

A brain aneurysm is an outpouching in an artery in the brain resulting from a defect in the artery wall, which may be exacerbated by age, high blood pressure, and genetic factors. Although the rupture of an aneurysm in the brain is a relatively infrequent type of stroke (about twenty thousand people per year in the United States), the results can be devastating: about one-third of those suffering from a ruptured brain aneurysm die before reaching the hospital, another one-third are permanently impaired (e.g., paralysis, loss of language function), and only one-third escape relatively intact neurologically. Clearly, optimizing the diagnosis of a brain aneurysm—ideally before it has ruptured—as well as the treatment should be of prime importance for the health-care system.

Until about twenty years ago, the definitive treatment of brain aneurysms, ruptured or unruptured, involved a neurosurgeon performing a craniotomy (opening the skull under general anesthesia) and placing a small metal clip across the base of the aneurysmal outpouching. Although usually this treatment cured the aneurysm from further bleeding (or the possibility of bleeding, if unruptured), a craniotomy to clip an aneurysm frequently required retracting portions of the brain to access the region of the aneurysm. The morbidity of such an operation, as well as the financial expense of the procedure and the postprocedure intensive care unit stay of several days or more, was considerable. A less invasive treatment for brain aneurysms would be a major advance.

Such an advance has occurred gradually over the past twenty years with the advent of interventional neuroradiology—radiologists trained in threading a small catheter up the femoral artery in the groin past the heart and up one of the two carotid or two vertebral arteries, which supply blood to the brain. At the tip of the catheter, there are small coils (and more recently, small cylindrical stents) that can be used to fill the offending aneurysm and cause blood to clot within it or wall it off from the parent artery. This endovascular technique avoids the craniotomy and manipulation of the brain necessary for clipping an aneurysm, and it has been shown to be significantly less expensive than clipping (despite the fact that the coils or stents for a single patient may cost thousands of dollars).

However, unless a neurosurgeon undertook the couple years of additional training necessary to become an endovascular neurosurgeon (similar to the training of the endovascular or interventional neuroradiologist), the neurosurgeon would not be in a position personally to choose to perform either (1) a craniotomy and clipping or (2) an endovascular (coil/stent) technique. Similarly, an interventional neuroradiologist would not be trained to perform a craniotomy. Thus a patient with a brain aneurysm would frequently be subjected to the treatment that his or her physician was in a position to perform and not necessarily the treatment that was best for the patient's particular brain aneurysm (in neurosurgical parlance, "clip versus coil").

Fortunately, over the past decade or so, major medical centers (usually affiliated with a medical school training both vascular neurosurgeons and endovascular neuroradiologists) have brought together their neurosurgery and neuroradiology departments to evaluate each patient with a brain aneurysm jointly so that the patient receives the optimal treatment. To be truly unbiased in the selection of clip versus coil treatment, the economic benefits to the neurosurgeon, the neuroradiologist, and the hospital (i.e., the medical institution as a whole) must be equitable in the clip versus coil debate.

Unfortunately, many smaller hospitals that have neurosurgeons on staff do not have an interventional neuroradiologist on staff to provide the endovascular option for a patient with a brain aneurysm. Although some neurosurgeons will transfer such a patient to an institution with both the clip and coil treatment options, the economic loss to both the neurosurgeon and the hospital (including the physicians staffing the intensive care unit, etc., that the patient would utilize during the pre- and postoperative stay) that results from such a transfer creates a powerful incentive for the clip option to be exercised. As skilled endovascular neuroradiologists become more widely available, this scenario is becoming somewhat less prevalent—but it is still not infrequent. Although guidelines can be promulgated for transfer of the brain aneurysm patient to an appropriately staffed medical center, unless such guidelines have "legal teeth" (i.e., significant financial or licensing penalties) they are unlikely to be very persuasive in changing the behavior of for-profit (and even nonprofit but economically challenged) hospitals—not to mention the behavior of fee-for-service neurosurgeons. As was seen in the last chapter regarding the skirting of EMTALA regulations in the interest of benefiting the economic bottom line (and not the patient's ultimate outcome), even regulations with serious penalties can be gamed by clever individuals and institutions (both physicians and medical administrators).

Surgery or Radiosurgery?

A similar turf war has arisen with the advent of radiosurgery for the treatment of certain tumors and blood vessel abnormalities in the brain and spinal cord, also over the past twenty to thirty years. Radiosurgery is a technique that uses a high dose of radiation focused very precisely on a small volume of tissue to destroy all cells within that volume while sparing the surrounding tissue. The similarity of radiosurgery and surgical excision in effect on a tumor (in the brain or elsewhere in the body) is captured in the trade names for two radiosurgery devices: the Gamma Knife and the CyberKnife.

Once radiosurgery devices became quite widely available—about twenty years ago—the neurosurgical literature clearly reflected the turf war that evolved in the treatment of certain brain tumors. The turf war involved most notably tumors that had spread to the brain from a primary site elsewhere in the body (metastatic brain tumors), meningiomas (tumors that arise from the tissue—the dura—surrounding the brain and spinal cord), and vestibular schwannomas (also known as acoustic neuromas—tumors located immediately inside the base of the skull at the level of the nerve for hearing, hence hearing loss is usually the initial complaint of the patient). Although tumors originating from brain tissue are relatively rare—occurring about as frequently as brain aneurysms (roughly twenty-five thousand patients per year in the United States)—metastatic brain tumors are at least five times as frequent (well over one hundred thousand patients per year) and more commonly detected now, thanks to increasingly sensitive MRI scanning techniques.

The turf war consisted of centers advocating surgical excision of metastatic brain tumors, meningiomas, and vestibular schwannomas vying with centers advocating radiosurgical treatment of these tumors—and supporting their choice with articles in peer-review journals. None of these publications were randomized, prospective in nature, and thus the conclusions of the authors on either side of the debate (surgical excision versus radiosurgery) more accurately reflected their particular bias than valid reasoning. To those of us who tried to approach the treatment of such patients with an unbiased eye, the publications debating the two treatment modalities verged on comedy; determining the optimal treatment for a given patient was not the goal of these publications, but rather vindication of the authors' chosen technique, either surgical excision or radiosurgery.

Fortunately, the company producing the Gamma Knife—Elekta—has from the device's inception required that any physician involved in radiosurgery treatment using the Gamma Knife must participate in a weeklong course in radiation biology, appropriate selection of patients to be treated, and the planning of treatment using the Gamma Knife. This includes both the neurosurgeon and the radiation oncologist who are involved in the patient's care. The other radiosurgery device manufacturers have not been so stringent on their requirements for physician training, nor have most hospitals. After all, if a hospital has invested several million dollars purchasing a radiosurgery device, it has a vested financial interest in seeing that as many radiosurgical procedures as possible are performed with that device—and the more neurosurgeons who are granted privileges to perform radiosurgery in that hospital, the larger the number of patients who are likely to undergo radiosurgical treatment.

Apart from this financial incentive for a hospital to encourage as many radiosurgical procedures to be performed as possible, there is a financial incentive for a neurosurgeon to consider surgical excision over radiosurgical treatment. The reimbursement to the neurosurgeon for performing a craniotomy to remove a brain tumor is two times (or more) as great as the reimbursement to the neurosurgeon for performing a radiosurgical treatment. Thus many neurosurgeons, to protect their own personal financial bottom line, are biased toward surgical excision rather than radiosurgical treatment. As a neurosurgeon who has treated many hundreds of patients with brain tumors—utilizing both surgical excision and radiosurgery—I recall only one patient (with a deep-seated but relatively large metastatic brain tumor) where either technique appeared equally safe and efficacious for that given patient. When all factors are included—patient age and medical condition, as well as tumor location, size, and type—virtually every patient is best treated by one technique or the other (and is not a good candidate for the other technique). Indeed, some patients can only be treated optimally by combined surgical excision *and* radiosurgical treatment (e.g., a patient with a meningioma too large for radiosurgical treatment alone but in an area of the brain where complete surgical excision is either impossible or overly risky, or a patient with several metastatic brain tumors, one of which is too large for radiosurgical treatment and thus requires surgical excision).

Ideally patients with tumors and other lesions in the brain and spinal cord would be evaluated and treated by a team of physicians with training in all the relevant treatment options—and without a financial incentive to favor one treatment over another. This clearly does not exist at present in the health-care system in the United States, yet it is essential for optimal patient care.

Can a Device Put a Doctor Out of a Job?

Some implanted medical devices clearly are both beneficial and cost-effective. Cardiac pacemakers fall into this category. Over the past ten to twenty years, two such implanted devices for disorders of the nervous system are deep brain stimulator (DBS) systems and vagus nerve stimulator (VNS) systems.

DBS was described briefly in chapter 9. DBS has proved over the past twenty years to be the most important advance in the treatment of Parkinson's disease since the discovery of dopamine (in the form of L-dopa, to cross the blood-brain barrier and thus effectively reach the brain) in the late 1960s. DBS requires surgical procedures to implant the electrode (or electrodes) into the appropriate region of the brain and to place the battery and microprocessor (which are together termed the pulse generator). The pulse generator is very similar to a cardiac pacemaker, and it is usually placed in the same subcutaneous position below the clavicle or collarbone. Parkinson's disease already afflicts at least one million people in the United States and is becoming more prevalent as people are living longer. Although new drugs to treat Parkinson's disease (and the use of stem cells to replace the deficiency in dopamine that is the hallmark of Parkinson's disease) are the subject of intense research efforts, no major treatment breakthroughs have occurred in over forty years. As the disease progresses, the drugs to treat Parkinson's disease typically become gradually less effective or they result in disabling side effects, such as dyskinesias (involuntary movements), usually within five years or so of diagnosis of the disease and initial drug treatment.

The implanted DBS hardware—an electrode in the brain and a pulse generator under the skin of the chest wall—costs nearly $20,000 for the typical bilateral (right and left hemisphere of the brain) placement. Despite this significant cost of the DBS device (plus well over twice that $20,000 in hospital charges for the surgery to implant the electrodes and the pulse generators), health-care insurance companies have consistently paid for the implantation of DBS in appropriately selected patients with advanced Parkinson's disease. This was true for several years even before the FDA had approved DBS for stimulation of the subthalamic nucleus in the brain for advanced Parkinson's disease in 2002. It is not that the health-care insurers were particularly humanitarian with regard to the benefits of DBS for the patient suffering from advanced Parkinson's disease—rather, they knew that DBS saved them money in the long run. The new medications for Parkinson's disease might cost up to $500 per month or more, since most Parkinson's disease patients are on more than one medication. Moreover, the patient could avoid an emergency room visit or an inpatient hospitalization (e.g., a broken hip or a head injury), because he or she was less likely to fall; these hospital visits quickly resulted in costs exceeding the costs of placing a DBS system.

Regarding epilepsy, about one out of every three patients with epilepsy is unable to have complete control of his or her seizures even with a combination of three or more of the available antiepileptic medications. Moreover, the side effects of these medications—most notably drowsiness and impaired thinking—can be significantly disabling, especially when more than one medication is taken. And, as with medications for Parkinson's disease, the expense of the medications for a given patient can easily run $500 or more per month. As with Parkinson's disease and DBS, several studies years ago documented the economic benefits of VNS placement in patients whose epilepsy has proven refractory to medications. The reasons are straightforward: (1) if the dose and/or number of medications can be reduced, the economic savings are substantial; (2) VNS can reduce not only the number but also the severity of the seizures in many patients, greatly reducing the number of emergency room visits and hospitalizations; (3) in a small percentage of patients (less than 10% in most series), the seizures can be completely controlled with VNS (usually with some antiepileptic medication[s] as well)—with a significant impact on the patient's ability to obtain and hold down a job, get a driver's license, and avoid dependence on social services. Indeed, as VNS is tried in patients more quickly once it is clear that medications alone are not curative (i.e., in patients—usually children or teenagers—who have had epilepsy for less than five years), the success rate of VNS in terms of either dramatic reduction in seizure frequency or complete control of seizures is significantly higher than in patients who have had refractory seizures for longer than five years (oftentimes the patients have had refractory seizures for decades).

Despite the economic and social quality-of-life incentives for both DBS and VNS, it is generally agreed that both DBS and VNS are much less commonly performed than they should be for optimal health care in the United States. The vast majority of neurosurgeons and neurologists who specialize in the evaluation and treatment of potential candidates for either DBS or VNS would like to be performing more of this type of treatment for patients who have not been successfully treated with less invasive techniques. In light of their cost-saving and quality-of-life benefits, why are DBS and VNS so underutilized? To a certain extent with DBS surgery, there is reticence on the part of some patients with Parkinson's disease to undergo a procedure invading the brain with electrodes given the relatively small chance of a possibly life-threatening intracranial hemorrhage or infection. This is less of a factor in VNS surgery, where the rate of a serious complication is very low in centers with experience in VNS surgery (which is performed on an outpatient basis).

The major reason for underutilization of both DBS for Parkinson's disease and VNS for epilepsy is the failure of patients who might be good candidates to be referred to a center with neurologists and neurosurgeons trained to evaluate prospective patients for these surgical treatments. Unfortunately, many primary care physicians are unaware of which of their patients might be a good candidate for one of these implanted devices. More surprisingly, many neurologists fall into the same category (i.e., they are unaware of those patients with Parkinson's disease or epilepsy who are likely to benefit from DBS or VNS, respectively). There appears to be a somewhat less innocent reason, however, than mere lack of knowledge. If one surveys either the publications that consider research on Parkinson's disease or on epilepsy or the proceedings of the national and international conferences for neurologists, the percentage of effort (in terms of numbers of scholarly papers published or presentations made) dedicated to either DBS or VNS is a fraction of what would be expected given the impact both DBS and VNS have made in the past decade on patients with Parkinson's disease and epilepsy, respectively.

One might think this situation of "neurologist with a pill" versus "neurosurgeon with a scalpel" is similar to debates on the relative merits of drugs versus surgery for coronary artery disease (cardiologist versus cardiac surgeon). However, the situation in the treatment options for advanced Parkinson's disease and refractory epilepsy is really very different. The patients with advanced Parkinson's disease or refractory epilepsy have exhausted all the pharmacologic options. DBS and VNS are not surgical substitutes for medications but rather a last-ditch attempt to improve the patient's quality of life after medications have failed to provide adequate treatment. Moreover, it is the rare patient with either advanced Parkinson's disease or refractory epilepsy who is able to forego medications entirely after either DBS or VNS; the majority of patients are able to only reduce the number of medications taken (or reduce the dose of a given medication), not eliminate medications entirely. Although patients who have undergone either DBS or VNS still need their neurologist for clinical care and medication follow-up for the rest of their life—just as if they had not undergone DBS or VNS—it seems to be difficult for many neurologists to realize that for some patients with Parkinson's disease or epilepsy, optimizing the patient's care requires a joint effort involving both the neurologist and the neurosurgeon. If more patients were appropriately referred for DBS and VNS, the neurologists would see their patient population expand as more people with these disorders are impressed by the positive outcome experienced by a friend, colleague, or relative with either Parkinson's disease or epilepsy.

Ironically, in the case of DBS and VNS, the for-profit health-care insurance companies have led the way in advocating for optimal patient care. The best treatment really is cheaper in the long run!

Changing the Turf from Crab Grass to Bermuda Grass

These three examples of turf wars have their basis in real (but short-term) economic benefit to the neurosurgeon (in the treatment of cerebral aneurysms and in the use of either surgical excision or radiosurgery in the treatment of brain tumors) and in perceived economic benefit to the neurologist (in the avoidance of DBS and VNS as treatments for their patients). All three illustrate the "zero-sum game" thinking that has pervaded physicians in the United States. Until the health-care system is configured so that the individual physician is motivated to consider the patient's medical outcome first and not the physician's own short-term economic benefit first (or worse still, misperception of short-term economic benefit), physicians will continue to be encouraged by "the system" to be constantly looking over their shoulder to see if other physicians are making incursions into their economic province.

In short, is health care an employment agency for physicians or a mechanism for optimizing the health of the populace?

Chapter 15: The Greenbacking of Medical/Surgical Societies

The professional medical and surgical societies of the physicians and surgeons in the United States were formed for the noble goals advocated in the Hippocratic Oath.

American Medical Association (AMA):

> Mission: To promote the art and science of medicine and the betterment of public health.
>
>> Core Values:
>> 1. Leadership
>> 2. Excellence
>> 3. Integrity and Ethical Behavior[48]

California Medical Association (CMA):

> Mission: Promoting the science and art of medicine, the care and well-being of patients, the protection of the public health, and the betterment of the medical profession.[49]

American College of Surgeons (ACS):

> Mission: The American College of Surgeons is dedicated to improving the care of the surgical patient and to safeguarding standards of care in an optimal and ethical practice environment.[50]

California Association of Neurological Surgeons (CANS):

Purpose: It shall be the purpose of this corporation:

— To promote and encourage the organization and professional association of duly licensed doctors of medicine in the State of California who are specializing in neurological surgery

— To promote in all respects the medical practice, continuing education, and advancement of the discipline of neurological surgery

— To promote scientific and professional exchange between members of this Association

— To maintain and strive constantly to improve the high quality of neurosurgical care for the people of the State of California

— To encourage rapid dissemination of knowledge concerning advances in neurosurgical techniques and diagnostic methods

— To promote in all respects through meetings, seminars, and publications the purposes of this Association

— To create a specialty medical society that can represent its membership in all matters of direct concern to them[51]

However, the medical and surgical societies are not ignorant of the economic aspects of medicine in the United States currently, nor are they immune from the lure of for-profit medicine tactics. Both the AMA and the CMA have created a political action committee (PAC) to sponsor the goals of their membership in Washington, DC, and Sacramento, California, respectively:

American Medical Association Political Action Committee (AMPAC):

AMPAC is the bipartisan political action committee of the American Medical Association. AMPAC's mission is to find and support candidates for congressional offices, whether it is a new candidate for office who will make physicians and patients a top priority, or a candidate running for reelection who has proven to be a friend of medicine.[52]

California Medical Association Political Action Committee (CALPAC):

Health care in California is highly regulated and legislated. As government and the insurance industry continue their quest to control health care, your clinical autonomy is in great jeopardy. Now more than ever, you need to fight to keep medical decisions in your well-trained hands. Fortunately, you do not have to wage the fight alone ...

CALPAC is a voluntary political organization that contributes to candidates for state and federal office who share our philosophy and vision of the future of medicine. Political law and CALPAC policy determines how your contribution to CALPAC is allocated. CMA will not favor or disadvantage anyone based on the amounts of or failure to make PAC contributions, nor will it affect your membership status with the CMA. Contributions to PAC's are voluntary and not limited to the suggested amounts.

Contributions are not deductible for state or federal income tax purposes.[53]

One of the primary mechanisms by which each professional society fulfills its mission is its annual meeting. The annual meeting is one of the major means by which the society educates its members (other means being educational courses, professional journals, etc.). As an example of how the focus of one society's annual meeting has changed, below are listed the presentations in the 1996 annual meeting of the California Association of Neurological Surgeons, followed by the presentations fifteen years later in the 2011 annual meeting. The two programs are listed in detail to facilitate the discussion that follows.

California Association of Neurological Surgeons Annual Meeting Program January 20–21, 1996:

Session I: Government and Neurosurgery

— Perspective of the President of a National Professional Organization
Sidney Tolchin, M.D., President,
American Association of Neurological Surgeons

— Perspective of the Speaker of the AMA House of Delegates
Richard Corlin, M.D.,
Speaker of the AMA House of Delegates

— The Political Perspective
Congressman William Thomas,
California 21st District

— California Advantage
Jack Lewin, M.D., Executive Vice President,
California Medical Association

Session II: Issues in the Changing Environment

— Investigational Drugs: Clinical Trials and Their Approval
>> Lawrence Marshall, M.D.,
>> California Association of Neurological Surgeons

— The Care of the Patient with Neural Trauma in California: "COBRA Plus"*
>> Thomas Hoyt, M.D.,
>> California Association of Neurological Surgeons

— Neuro Patients and the Distribution of Neurologists
>> Matthew Menken, M.D., Chairman,
>> World Federation of Neurology

— Neuro Patients and the Distribution of Neurological Surgeons
>> Martin Weiss, M.D.,
>> California Association of Neurological Surgeons

— Socioeconomic Issues in Neurology and Neurosurgery in Relation to the National Match**
>> Byron C. Pevehouse, M.D.,
>> California Association of Neurological Surgeons

---

* COBRA (Consolidated Omnibus Budget Reconciliation Act of 1985); "The Consolidated Omnibus Budget Reconciliation Act (COBRA) gives workers and their families who lose their health benefits the right to choose to continue group health benefits provided by their group health plan for limited periods of time under certain circumstances such as voluntary or involuntary job loss, reduction in the hours worked, transition between jobs, death, divorce, and other life events."[55]
** The [Residency] Match: "The NRMP Main Match provides an impartial venue for matching applicants' preferences for residency positions with program directors' preferences for applicants. Each year approximately 16,000 US allopathic medical school seniors and 15,000 graduates of osteopathic, Canadian, or foreign medical schools compete for approximately 24,000 residency positions."[56]

Session III: Responding to a Changing Environment

— AANS [American Association of Neurological Surgeons]
Guidelines for the Treatment of Head Injury
Randall M. Chestnut, M.D.,
Chief of Neurosurgical Services,
San Francisco General Hospital

— Patient Outcomes in an Individual Neurosurgical Practice
Randall W. Smith, M.D., President,
California Association of Neurological Surgeons

— State Action Exemption
George Koenig, M.D.,
California Association of Neurological Surgeons

— The Care of the Neurosurgical Patient: Projections into
Managed Care
John Kusske, M.D.,
California Association of Neurological Surgeons

— CANS View on Overhead Expenses
John Bonner, M.D.,
California Association of Neurological Surgeons

— Guidelines for the Treatment of the Patient with Back
Injury
DeWitt Gifford, M.D.,
California Association of Neurological Surgeons

California Association of Neurological Surgeons Annual Meeting Program
January 15–16, 2011:

Session I: The Future of Your Neurosurgical Practice After Health
Care Reform

— The Impact of Federal Health Care Legislation on
Hospitals and Neurosurgeons in California
Anne McLeod,
Senior Vice President of Health Policy,
California Hospital Association

— New Models of Care under Health Care Reform
John Jenrette, M.D.,
Chief Executive & Medical Officer,
Sharp Community Medical Group, San Diego

— Federal and State Law: Its Effect on Your Future Practice
Gary Spradling, Attorney,
Duckor Spradling Metzger & Wynne

— Locum Tenens***
Therus C. Kolff, M.D.;
Duane B. Gainsburg, M.D.;
John G. Hayes, Weatherby Locums

— Medical Device Distributorship Model
Angela Carlson, President,
Alliance Surgical Distributors

*** Locum tenens: "a physician who is contracted to work on a temporary basis to
fill in for a vacancy, vacation, or extended leave."[57]

— Gain Sharing with Hospitals
> Matthew Cutler, Chief Executive Officer,
> Select Health Care Solutions

— Leverage Your Medical Expertise as an Expert Witness
> Rosalie Hamilton,
> Expert Witness Marketing Consultant,
> Expert Communications

— The Challenge of the New Health Care Legislation to Academic Neurosurgery
> Bob Carter, M.D., Chief of Neurosurgery,
> University of San Diego Medical Center

Session II: Electronic Health Records (EHR)

— Come and listen to a general overview from a major EHR vendor who will provide some important information about what to consider before purchasing a system. Individual software packages will not be compared in this discussion ... vendors will be available at exhibit tables should you wish to ask specific questions or if you want to schedule an appointment for a demonstration.
> Presented by Allscripts
> ["Allscripts is recognized industry-wide as a
> provider of leading health care software solutions"
> —Allscripts website <www.allscripts.com>][54]

Of the fifteen presentations at the 1996 CANS annual meeting, all but one were by practicing physicians (the one exception being a California congressman). Although some of the presentations considered legislative and legal aspects of neurosurgical care, the majority considered topics directly or indirectly related to the clinical care of neurosurgical patients.

None of the presentations could be considered to have the goal of benefiting the neurosurgeon's personal financial gain.

Of the nine presentations in the 2011 CANS annual meeting, only one was solely by a practicing physician. One other presentation was by a physician in an administrative role (the CEO of the Sharp Community Medical Group), and another presentation was partly by practicing physicians (but as advocates of *locum tenens* positions for neurosurgeons). Several presentations considered the legal and financial aspects of joint ventures (e.g., physician-managed hospitals and surgery centers, joint ventures like MRI and radiosurgery centers, and medical device distributorships). All of these presentations, including those on *locum tenens* positions for neurosurgeons and expert witness activities, were primarily aimed at augmenting the individual neurosurgeon's economic situation or financial bottom line. Finally, the entire three-hour session on day two was a presentation by an electronic medical record vendor.

The shift in focus of the California Association of Neurological Surgeons annual meeting from 1996 to 2011 is quite astounding. In 2011, none of the presentations considered actual clinical care of the neurosurgical patient, whereas in 1996 the majority of the presentations were clinically focused and presented by practicing neurosurgeons. Virtually the entire 2011 CANS annual meeting was focused on improving the "financial health" of the neurosurgeon rather than improving the "neurosurgical health" of the patient.

Is this the direction that health care in the United States should be taking?

Chapter 16: Where Has All the Money Gone?
Wealthy Middlemen in Medical Devices

There are many reasons why health care in the United States is consuming upward of 20% of the GDP. Health care has become the country's "cash cow"; the huge profits and extravagant reimbursements (salaries, bonuses, etc.) of upper-level management personnel in the health insurance industry are testaments to that. However, there are many others who are profiting handsomely, without overall benefit to the health of the populace. One example from the 2011 meeting of the California Association of Neurological Surgeons discussed in the previous chapter is illustrative:

> — Medical Device Distributorship Model
>> Angela Carlson, President,
>> Alliance Surgical Distributors

Alliance Surgical Products was formed in 2007 by four physicians in Southern California (discussed in an article in *Press-Enterprise*, Riverside, California, October 1, 2009).[58] The group was started by an orthopedic surgeon who became incensed at soaring health-care costs, specifically the cost of joint and spine implants to hospitals where joint replacement and spinal hardware surgery is performed. This impression was supported by a 2006 study in the *Journal of Bone and Joint Surgery* that presented data comparing joint replacement surgery costs in the United States in 1994 and 2006.[59] While hospital profit declined 92% and surgeon reimbursement declined 39% during that period, the cost of implants increased 171%.

The purpose of Alliance Surgical Products is simple: replace the middleman (or middlemen) distributorships between the implant manufacturer and the purchaser (the hospital) with a surgeon-owned distributorship. Although the free market is supposed to keep the cost to the consumer (in this case, the hospital purchasing the implant) low, in reality the middlemen distributors manage to make a handsome profit. Just how large this profit is proved to be quite staggering.

From May 2006 through May 2008, the surgeon-owned company distributed implants to three hospitals for four common implant procedures: total knee replacement, total hip replacement, posterior lumbar spine (pedicle screw) instrumentation, and anterior cervical spine (plate) instrumentation. There were 544 total cases: 217 total joint replacements and 327 spinal instrumentations. The cost of these 544 implants to the hospitals was compared with the cost of the average contracted price (not the list price) to the hospitals with the distributor middlemen:

Average Distributorship Contract Price	Surgeon-Owned Distributorship Price
$3,099,192	$2,058,217

The savings over this two-year period to the three hospitals on the 544 implants was $1,040,975—a 34% savings. Moreover, each of the four physicians managed to make a six-figure personal profit on this arrangement.

A 34% profit is enormous, and no doubt there are many other examples of huge profits in the health-care industry (the health insurance and pharmaceutical companies come to mind). Unlike most industries (from cars to apparel to computers), where the consumer can seek a cheaper competitor, health care in the United States is a huge monolith with little true competition. One might compare it with the banking industry, where exorbitant banking fees and interest rates become standardized across all major banks. In health care, one's only option—increasingly exercised by a minority of the populace—is to seek health care outside the United States (e.g., the medical tourism industry in Mexico and Thailand). However, going to Bangkok for one's annual physical exam or the flu or a urinary tract infection scarcely makes sense.

Like so many people in the general population whose obesity is becoming an increasing factor in the deteriorating health of the nation as a whole, the waste (unnecessary expense) in the health-care industry is a major factor in our declining health statistics in the United States.

Perhaps it is time to put the "health-care cash cow" on a serious diet!

Chapter 17: Medical Response to Disasters:
World-Style vs. USA-Style

The overarching organization for neurosurgery worldwide is the World Federation of Neurosurgical Societies (WFNS). It consists not of individual neurosurgeon members, but of the neurosurgical societies of countries on all six continents (126 neurosurgical societies in all). There are regional neurosurgical societies within the WFNS, such as the European Association of Neurosurgical Societies and the Federation of Latin American Neurosurgical Societies.[60]

In the aftermath of the devastating earthquakes in Haiti and Chile in early 2010, two committees of the WFNS (Education & Training Committee and International Initiatives Committee) began discussing how neurosurgery worldwide could improve our medical response to disasters, such as earthquakes, tsunamis, and terrorist attacks. It is indicative of the importance of improving our medical response to disasters that the Young Neurosurgeons' Forum of the WFNS—headed by a young neurosurgeon in Nigeria, Muhammad Raji Mahmud—selected the topic "neurosurgical response to disasters" for their first online teleconference for neurosurgeons worldwide in January 2011. The devastating earthquake/tsunami in Japan in March 2011 and others since then have emphasized the need for improved medical response to disasters in both developing and developed countries.

Although improving neurosurgical response to disasters has been considered formally by the WFNS for less than two years, it is bringing together ideas and individuals from various medical organizations worldwide to address improved medical care in the critical first hours and days after a disaster strikes; these include military medical response teams and programs, government health ministries (e.g., Chile), other medical organizations relevant to disaster response worldwide, and companies producing relevant products (e.g., telemedicine [Cisco Systems], portable CT scanners [NeuroLogica], and video equipment for remote surgical assisting [Vigilent Telesystems]).

One example of an effort to improve health care worldwide is the Pan-African E-Network Project initiated by the government of India's Ministry of External Affairs. The Indian government selected the Apollo Telemedicine Networking Foundation (ATNF) to provide medical teleconsultations and medical education telecourses; these telemedicine activities now reach fifty medical centers across twenty-nine African nations. Comprised of over fifty hospitals throughout India and in many nearby countries, the Apollo Hospitals Group has developed the largest multispecialty telemedicine network in South Asia. The president of the ATNF is Krishnan Ganapathy, a neurosurgeon in Chennai, India—home of the Apollo Hospitals Group—who has had a long-standing dedication to telemedicine for the benefit of both India and neighboring developing countries.

The effect of the Pan-African E-Network Project and the ATNF on health care for broad segments of the underserved populations throughout Africa cannot be overestimated. The fact that the Indian government and the Apollo Hospitals Group have had the foresight to address the health-care needs not only of its own population but those of its nearby (and not so nearby, in the case of Africa) neighbors is evidence of a humanitarian concern that Hippocrates would certainly endorse. The dedication and ingenuity of Dr. Ganapathy and colleagues in India, Africa, and elsewhere—achieving remarkable goals with limited resources—is a model that we in the United States might learn from.

In the United States, there are two national neurosurgical societies: the American Association of Neurological Surgeons (AANS) and the Congress of Neurological Surgeons (CNS). The AANS was formed in 1931 as the Harvey Cushing Society—in honor of Harvey Cushing, who was one of the world's most innovative neurosurgeons in the early twentieth century. The CNS was formed in 1951 by a group of younger neurosurgeons who felt constrained by the more senior AANS; the CNS in its early years emphasized neurosurgical education and research over the administrative and economic aspects of neurosurgery in particular and medicine in general. Over the years, the distinction between the AANS and the CNS has become blurred; one society has its annual meeting in the spring, the other in the fall—and if names and logos were removed, a participant might have difficulty telling which society's meeting was being attended.

Both of the societies have a monthly scholarly journal in which peer-reviewed clinical and research reports are presented. Both societies also have a quarterly publication—specifically aimed at their neurosurgeon membership—which presents information on various aspects of medicine in general and neurosurgery in particular, including administrative and economic issues. Thus when I perused the Fall 2011 issue of *Congress Quarterly* (the CNS publication), I should not have been surprised by the content of an article entitled "Significant Threat … Rapid Response."[61] Having been involved in the WFNS Neurosurgical Response to Disasters project, I was biased into expecting perhaps an update on neurotrauma programs in the United States. My naïveté is readily exposed by a quote from this article:

> The profession of Neurosurgery and care of our patients face constant threats. While these threats are numerous, perhaps none is more potentially damaging than that of the limitation of access to care brought about by adverse reimbursement policy decisions. To address these threats, organized neurosurgery must engage a team of highly skilled surgeons to respond to reviews and proposed policy changes. Moreover, the response must be rapid.
>
> To this end, the AANS/CNS Section on Disorders of the Spine and Peripheral Nerves has created a "Rapid Response Team." This group of unsung heroes is composed of experts in reading and deciphering policy, coding and reimbursement, clinical research, and evidence-based medicine. This team … has been developed to quickly address these threats to the practice of Neurosurgery and care of our patients identified by leadership and members.

Activities of the team may consist of the reviewing and reporting of similar policy responses, reviewing recent evidence, evidence-based medicine reports and precedent, as well as outlining any legal ramifications. A summary is created by the team, vetted by leadership, and submitted back to the policy provider, often a governmental entity or private insurer. This process often takes two to six weeks to fully review a threat, create a document, vet it through leadership and return it to the requesting organization.

[The] group is made up completely of surgeon volunteers facing a frequently daunting task. Third-party payers are under considerable liability regarding policy decisions that affect patient care. To this end, payers have assembled groups of experts in many fields such as law, policy, and evidence-based medicine. In order to address adverse policies and protect our patients, organized neurosurgery must therefore assemble its own group of policy experts trained to draw upon their specific knowledge of neurosurgery ... These rapid yet comprehensive responses are crucial to ensure our patients have access to the best treatments available and moreover to ensure physicians are not forced to limit patient care or leave their practices due to declining reimbursement.[61]

Perhaps the most telling phrase is the last, "moreover to ensure physicians are not forced to limit patient care or leave their practices due to declining reimbursement." Not only have neurosurgeons in the United States been forced to develop their own "rapid response teams" for financial issues, other organizations have been created with the sole purpose of improving a physician's financial bottom line. For example, the San Jose Surgical Society—a professional society of surgeons in the San Jose, California, area—had Ed Norwood (president of ERN/The National Council of Reimbursement Advocacy) as the speaker at their semiannual dinner meeting in May 2011. The purpose of ERN/NCRA is summarized in their vision statement:

ERN/NCRA Vision: ERN/NCRA ... will be the undisputable industry leader in reimbursement advocacy as measured by provider membership, case overturns, payer corrective action plans, and public policy reform. We will become a trusted name in health care compliance and an authority in administrative laws that govern the health care delivery process, relate to timely reimbursement, and prevent improper denials.[62]

Did this meeting have anything to do with the care of patients in San Jose with surgical health problems? Or did the society devote one of their two annual dinner meetings solely to the financial health of their individual practices?

Our neurosurgery colleagues in India are using the latest technology for telemedicine to bring state-of-the-art medicine to both rural India and much of Africa—with very limited resources. The WFNS—led by their Young Neurosurgeons' Forum—is dedicating increasing resources to the improvement of medical response to disasters worldwide (among many other issues affecting neurosurgical care around the world that the WFNS is concerned with). Neurosurgeons in the United States are now having to develop rapid response teams—not for medical care issues, but rather to address the financial and administrative issues that are sapping the energy and initiative from a medical specialty previously known for its innovative ideas and techniques: neurosurgery.

Were they to confront today's health care USA-style, I suspect both Hippocrates and Harvey Cushing would be turning over in their graves ...

Part IV

Healing American Medicine—What Should the Doctor Order?

Chapter 18: "Strike!" California's Medical Injury Compensation Reform Act of 1975 (MICRA)

In the decade preceding 1975, the number of medical malpractice claims in California doubled and the dollar amounts awarded in judgments or settlements increased tenfold. Thus by 1975, medical malpractice insurance companies has decided that:

> That year [1975] two malpractice insurance companies made major announcements: one notified 2,000 Southern California physicians that their malpractice insurance would not be renewed, and the other notified 4,000 Northern California physicians that their premiums would increase by 380 percent. These companies had determined that the California medical malpractice insurance market had become too risky and unstable for financially sound underwriting.[63]

These malpractice insurance changes were to take effect on May 1, 1975. The California Medical Association website describes what happened:

> Many medical physicians had four choices, none of them acceptable: raise fees and make medical care unaffordable for many patients, drop their professional liability insurance coverage, leave the state, or quit practicing medicine.

Newspaper headlines reflected the extent of the problem:

"New Bay Area Crisis in Medical Care: Doctors Might Halt Practice," *San Francisco Chronicle*, 1/31/75

119

"Doctors Face Insurance Crisis—May Affect 8,000 in Southland," *Los Angeles Times*, 2/22/75

"Insurance Rates Peril Medical Care," *San Jose Mercury News*, 2/23/75

As their premiums more than tripled, anesthesiologists and surgeons in the (San Francisco) Bay Area and other parts of Northern California began a walkout, refusing to handle any patients except those in imminent danger of death. Some hospitals agreed to pay premiums for anesthesiologists and some physicians agreed to work emergency cases without pay. Throughout the winter and spring of 1975, the crisis continued to escalate as the May 1 rate increase approached ...

On May 13, 1975, CMA led more than 800 physicians, nurses, lab technicians and hospital personnel in a Capitol rally calling on Gov. Edmund G. "Jerry" Brown, Jr., to convene a special session of the Legislature to deal with the crisis. Three days later, on May 16, Brown yielded, issuing a proclamation for a special session that began on May 19. Negotiations and legislative hearings that involved CMA and other health care providers, the insurance industry and trial lawyers continued until September 11, when the Legislature passed AB 1XX, a collection of statutes that is now known as the Malpractice Insurance Compensation Reform Act (MICRA). Governor Brown signed the CMA-supported bill on September 23, 1975, and MICRA today remains the model for national medical liability tort reform ...

Passage of MICRA was only the first step. Lawsuits challenging the constitutionality of MICRA weaved their way through the judicial system until 1985, when the California Supreme Court upheld its constitutionality with the following comments:

In enacting MICRA, the Legislature was acting in a situation in which it had found that the rising cost of medical malpractice insurance was posing serious problems for the health care system in California, threatening to curtail the availability of medical care in some parts of the state and creating the very real possibility that many doctors would practice without insurance, leaving patients who might be injured by such doctors with the prospect of uncollectible judgments. In attempting to reduce the cost of medical malpractice insurance in MICRA, the Legislature enacted a variety of provisions affecting doctors, insurance companies and malpractice plaintiffs. [The limitation on recoverable noneconomic damages] is, of course, one of the provisions which made changes in existing tort rules in an attempt to reduce the cost of medical malpractice litigation, and thereby restrain the increase in medical malpractice insurance premiums. It appears obvious that this section—by placing a ceiling of $250,000 on the recovery of noneconomic damages—is rationally related to the objective of reducing the costs of malpractice defendants and their insurers.

The California Supreme Court decision was appealed to the US Supreme Court, which, on October 15, 1985, declined to review the case, "for want of a substantial federal question." Thus, 10 years after passage, the question of MICRA's constitutionality finally was settled law.[64]

MICRA would not have come about in California—or certainly not have come about as quickly as it did during the summer of 1975—were it not for the physicians in Northern California having gone on strike for all but emergency medical care. Many other professions, from trade guilds to teachers, have used a strike as a means of calling attention to an intolerable situation. The strike by physicians that brought about MICRA sets a precedent that, although not to be exercised except in extreme medical duress, may be the only way in which progress to true health-care reform can be implemented.

Chapter 19: Global Medical Knowledge, Local Medical Implementation: Predictive, Preventive, and Personalized Medicine

Health-care reform will undoubtedly benefit from both high-tech and low-tech advances. On the high-tech end, perhaps the greatest contribution will come from our evolving knowledge of genomics. With the initial draft of the Human Genome Project in 2000, the twenty thousand–plus genes that make up the human genome were mapped, and research projects on the benefits of genomics for predicting and treating medical disorders were initiated.

That genomics will make a very significant impact on improving health care is not in doubt. Respected organizations like the Institute of Medicine (IOM) have begun sponsoring workshops on genomics, such as the IOM Roundtable on Translating Genomic-Based Research for Health ("Integrating Large-Scale Genomic Information into Clinical Practice") held on July 19, 2011. Many academic medical centers have created genomics medicine institutes, such as the University of California, San Diego, Institute for Genomic Medicine and the Cleveland Clinic Foundation Genomic Medicine Institute. Even nonacademic medical centers have begun to educate their physicians and their patients about the impact genomics will have on health care, as in the case of the Genomic Medicine Institute at El Camino Hospital in the San Francisco Bay Area.

Moreover, for-profit companies have not missed the opportunity to benefit financially from providing genetic information direct to "consumers" (i.e., patients). For example, 23andMe, Inc. (Mountain View, California) has a Personal Genome Service (PGS), which advertises:

"Get to know your DNA. All it takes is a little bit of spit."[65]

One merely sends 23andMe a saliva sample in a test tube, and six to eight weeks later one can review the genetic data online. However, 23andMe is very careful to describe the limitations of their service in their "Risks and Considerations Regarding 23andMe Services." Since 23andMe sequences only part of one's genome, it may miss variations that are of significance. Genetic testing services, on the other hand, more thoroughly investigate particular genes. To make an accurate diagnosis, additional information (e.g., personal health, family history) is needed and must be interpreted, together with the genetic information provided by 23andMe, by one's personal physician or a genetics expert.

23andMe has constructed a business model that more closely resembles the software industry than most other examples of health-care diagnosis and delivery. The entire relationship is conducted online or by mail, without interpretation of the findings or quality controls in case of computer error and misdiagnosis. And like the software industry, 23andMe has a guaranteed revenue stream in that each new upgrade (advance in the genome analysis technology) represents an additional charge to a patient/customer if he/she wishes to be kept up to date on the 23andMe platform. Also, a special sample collection kit for young children is available for an additional charge, so the whole family can experience the 23andMe service.

Further evidence that 23andMe is concerned more with profits than patients comes from a recent event with potential legal consequences. 23andMe appears to be using patients' genetic data to create patents for the company, without clear consent from their patients/consumers. The following quote from Pascal Borry, professor of bioethics at the University of Leuven in Belgium, summarizes the problem with assuming a consumer is automatically a research subject without obtaining specific consent for the use of genetic data for patent purposes:

There is nothing wrong [with 23andMe] using the direct-to-consumer genetic testing model for creating business revenues, but this conflicts with the transparent, science-driven image 23andMe has been creating of its research objectives. Consumers have been misled in that regard, and saying that [permission] was in the informed consent [that customers signed] is not sufficient.[66]

23andMe takes all major credit cards and ships to over fifty countries, and naturally you can offer a prepaid subscription for your family and friends. What better way to celebrate a loved one's birthday than to provide them the means to find out two months later that they have an incurable disease? Just make certain you forward them a copy of the 23andMe "Terms of Service" (which is nearly nine thousand words long).

The point of my somewhat cynical view is that if a group like 23andMe were truly interested in improving health care for all rather than maximizing its short-term profits, the company would have spent their resources to improve genotyping techniques and/or to educate physicians regarding the potential benefits of genotyping. There is perhaps a parallel with the primary care physician versus the hospitalist models: 23andMe has no obligation to the patient once the credit card has been charged and the results made available online, whereas the patient's physician (if he/she was better educated regarding genotyping and had access to more accurate/extensive genotyping results) is obligated to use that information to influence the patient's health care in a positive direction.

Predictive, Preventive, and Personalized Medicine—Not Just a European Union

A more comprehensive approach to the use of high-tech medicine for improved health care is provided by the European Association for Predictive, Preventive, and Personalized Medicine (EPMA). The EPMA is a consortium of physicians and medical researchers with institutional, governmental, and industry participants, not only from European Union (EU) countries, but also with representatives from as far away as Japan and Taiwan (more than forty countries in all). In addition to Institutional Members (primarily medical universities such as Charité Medical University in Berlin and the Medical University of Vienna), the EPMA has Academic and Industrial Advisory Boards:

Academic—experts in genomics, biotechnology and its commercialization, health care policy

Industrial—representatives from the Bracco Group (Italy), diaDexus (USA), Randox (UK), and Springer Medicine (The Netherlands)[67,68]

In the less than four years since its inception in November 2008, the EPMA has made remarkable progress:

2009: publication of *Predictive Diagnostics and Personalized Treatment: Dream or Reality?* Ed: O. Golubnitschaja, Nova Biomedical Books, New York

2010: publication of the *EPMA Journal*, four volumes per year, Springer Medical, Dordrecht

2011: First EPMA World Congress, Bonn, September 15–18

2012: publication of the book series *Advances in Predictive, Preventive, and Personalized Medicine*, four books per year, Springer Medical, Dordrecht[78]

The First EPMA World Congress, held September 2011, was notable for bringing together participants from forty-four countries. To quote from the abstract of the EPMA World Congress summary document:

European strategies related to PPPM [Predictive, Preventive, and Personalized Medicine] have been discussed in specialized sessions dedicated to:

— Health care in overview across the globe
— Collaboration with global organizations
— Granting strategies in PPPM

- Education in PPPM
- Patient needs
- Targeted prevention
- PPPM in reproductive medicine & pediatrics
- PPPM in diabetes care
- PPPM in neurodegenerative diseases
- PPPM in cancer
- PPPM in cardiovascular diseases
- Innovative PPPM-centers
- Biomarker validation and standards
- Patient-specific modeling and bioinformatics in PPPM
- PPPM-related bio-preservation, bio-banking & ethics

EPMA "expert recommendations" will be presented to Ministries of Health of forty-four contributing countries, partner societies, associations, funding agencies, and global organizations that participated in the congress. Full analysis of the outcomes will be provided during the next EPMA World Congress in September 2013.[67]

One should be encouraged by the forward-looking, eclectic, cross-disciplinary, and results-centered (rather than profits-centered) approach advocated by the EPMA. One section of the EPMA being developed is dedicated to PPPM economics:

The [economics] section will be dedicated to the economic and commercial aspects of PPPM. The goals and tasks of the section are considered to be as follows:

- Initiation of economic studies able to demonstrate the value of PPPM to society
- Supporting researchers in finding partners for effective development of PPPM-related scientific projects, with a clear focus on application

— Encouraging researchers to start their own companies with the midterm goal to take their PPPM projects to market
— Providing advice on how to access public and private funds[67]

By combining the resources of academia, industry, and public and private agencies in the EU countries and beyond (forty-four countries to date), the EPMA appears to be in a much stronger position to have a positive impact on health care than a fragmented, individualistic approach that relies upon the interests of for-profit companies. We saw in chapter 11 (and elsewhere) that when for-profit companies are left to their own motives (i.e., to maximize profit in the short run), the health care of the population in general is more likely to suffer than to benefit.

Patient-Centered Medical Home versus Profit-Centered Medical Industry

The EPMA exemplifies the high-tech, and in some aspects "global" (both geographically and comprehensively), approach to improving health care. But where the rubber hits the road is in the doctor–patient relationship, where the collective health-care knowledge is applied to the particular patient's health-care situation. As is typical for the reporting of health-care issues in the United States, the following quote outlines the problem in stark economic terms:

A volume-oriented fee-for-service reimbursement system with relatively low reimbursement rates when compared to specialists has perpetuated a dysfunctional primary care system that rewards quantity over quality ... This deeply flawed system has led to per capita costs nearly twice that of the next most expensive industrialized country with serious deficiencies in the quality of outpatient care ... The patient-centered medical home (PCMH) has been touted as a model for delivery system reform that may address many of these market failures and inefficiencies, and potentially rescue primary care from possible extinction.[69]

The PCMH model for health-care delivery was initially proposed by the American Academy of Pediatrics (AAP) more than forty years ago. In 2007, the AAP—together with the American Academy of Family Physicians (AAFP), the American College of Physicians (ACP), and the American Osteopathic Association (AOA), comprising over 330,000 physicians in all—presented their "Joint Principles of the Patient-Centered Medical Home." In 2010–2011, the AAFP, AAP, ACP, and AOA published "Guidelines for Patient-Centered Medical Home (PCMH) Recognition and Accreditation Programs" as well as "Joint Principles for the Medical Education of Physicians as Preparation for Practice in the Patient-Centered Medical Home."

The essence of the PCMH model is revealed in the basic principles put forth by the AAP, AAFP, ACP, and AOA, the most salient of which are summarized as follows:

1. Every patient (child or adult) has a personal physician with whom there is continuous and comprehensive care.
2. The personal physician directs a team of health-care professionals who are responsible collectively for the ongoing care of the patient.
3. The personal physician is responsible for coordinating the patient's care in all settings and conditions—acute and chronic care, preventive care, and end of life care.
4. The patient's care is coordinated or integrated across all aspects of the health-care delivery system—community-based services, home health agencies, general medical and subspecialty hospital care, and nursing homes.
5. Information technology such as electronic health records are used to guarantee prompt, accurate, and cost-effective health care.
6. Resources are made available for linguistically and culturally appropriate health care.[70]

The PCMH concept has been especially prominent in implementation since the National Committee for Quality Assurance (NCQA) has developed standards for implementing and assessing the PCMH in clinical settings. The NCQA is a private, not-for-profit 501(c)(3) organization whose principal sponsors include foundations (The California Endowment and The Commonwealth Fund) and drug companies ($250,000 or more per year from Boerhringer-Ingelheim, Merck, and McNeil Pediatrics Division of Ortho-McNeil-Janssen Pharmaceuticals).

The NCQA PCMH 2011 evaluation program for PCMH sites includes six standards, twenty-seven elements, and on hundred forty-nine factors.[71] The six standards are: (1) enhance access and continuity; (2) identify and manage patient populations; (3) plan and manage care; (4) provide self-care and community support; (5) track and coordinate care; (6) measure and improve performance. These six standards are mapped into the PCMH 2011 goals: (1) increase patient-centeredness; (2) align requirements with processes that improve quality and eliminate waste; (3) increase emphasis on patient feedback; (4) enhance the use of clinical performance measures; (5) integrate behaviors affecting health, mental health, and substance abuse; (6) enhance coordination of care.

The essence of the PCMH concept is expressed in the following quote by Margaret E. O'Kane, president of NCQA:

"The Patient-Centered Medical Home is a model of twenty-first century primary care that combines access, teamwork, and technology to deliver quality care and improve health."[72]

The growth of the NCQA PCMH program has been impressive, from 28 sites and 214 clinicians in December 2008 to 1,506 sites and 7,676 clinicians in December 2010; the NCQA website reported 3,060 sites as of December 2011. However, PCMH demonstration projects in the United States are much broader in number than those following the NCQA evaluation program. One nationwide survey of PCMH demonstration projects interviewed twenty-six projects that included over fourteen thousand physicians caring for nearly five million patients.[68] Another recent review considered over two hundred publications (journal articles, books, and reports) on PCMH and produced the following conclusion:

"A combination of fee-for-service, case management fees, and quality outcome incentives effectively drive higher standards in patient experience and outcomes [with medical homes]."[73]

A second quote from the same article presents the issue bluntly when one considers health care as "cost center" and not as a basic human right of citizenship (i.e., the right to life of the Declaration of Independence):

"Medical practices are business entities. Rewards for change must exceed the cost of change."[73]

Another review of PCMH demonstration sites offers a somewhat more humanitarian assessment of the motivation for PCMH. These authors argue for universal PCMH availability, with the principal goal of improving health care and the secondary goal of health-care payment reform. Since primary care physician groups are unlikely to be able to finance the transformation to PCMH (in hopes of recovering the expense in the future), it will be necessary to have funding from various stakeholders (e.g., federal, state, and local governments; the medical insurance industry; and health-care systems). Transparency in negotiating the transformation to the PCMH is essential to avoid hidden agendas. The conclusion of the article is quite to the point:

Primary care, like healthy food, works best at a local and personal level. What is waste on an assembly line is not necessarily waste in a healing relationship; allow for appropriate variability. Stewarding patients toward healthier lives is a deliberate process—stewarding practices toward health and toward becoming a PCMH is also.[74]

It is intriguing that the principal supporters of the profit-centered, "big business" health-care system in the United States at present are those who claim to want the country to return to the principles of the Constitution that our forefathers intended the country to follow. As noted in the introduction, the first inalienable right in the Declaration of Independence is the right to life. As presented throughout this volume, our present system of health-care delivery in the United States puts health-care economics above health care itself. Ironically—taken to the extreme—for-profit medicine could be worse than no health-care system at all.

Those who chant "socialized medicine" as a mantra to be avoided at all costs (pun intended) should heartily embrace the concepts of for-profit organ donation, for-profit abortions, and for-profit use of embryonic stem cells.

Chapter 20: "Go West, Young Doctor; Go East, Young Doctor; Go Anywhere Outside the United States, Young Doctor!"

Health Care in Developed Countries Worldwide

A large study funded primarily by the Commonwealth Fund and published in 2007 surveyed the health-care experiences of adults in seven countries: Australia, New Zealand, Canada, Germany, the Netherlands, the United Kingdom, and the United States.[74] Representative samples of adults age eighteen and older were interviewed by telephone for an average of seventeen minutes each, the approximate numbers of adults interviewed in each country being Australia and New Zealand (1,000); Germany, the Netherlands, and the United Kingdom (1,500); the United States (2,500); and Canada (3,000).

The results—the opinions of the adults interviewed in the seven countries—are given in seven tables (referred to as "exhibits" in the publication):

— Overview: Health Spending and Insurance Systems in Seven Countries (Australia, Canada, Germany, the Netherlands, New Zealand, the United Kingdom, and the United States), 2007
— Health System Views, Confidence, and Cost
— Patients' Reports of Primary Care Relationship and Accessibility
— Primary Care Access and Hospital Emergency Room Use

132

— Doctor–Patient Communication and Care Coordination
— Experiences of Patients with Chronic Conditions
— Medical, Medication, and Lab Errors[75]

The exhibits are quite lengthy and not readily summarized across the seven countries. However, a summary of the exhibit 1 (Overview of Health Spending and Insurance Systems in Seven Countries [Australia, Canada, Germany, the Netherlands, New Zealand, the United Kingdom, and the United States], 2007) is worthy of consideration here. Overall health spending per capita was more than twice as high in the United States ($6,697) than in the next highest spending country (Canada: $3,326). In percent of GDP spent on health care, the United States at 16% was 50% higher than the next highest country (Germany: 10.7%). The country with the lowest health spending in terms of GDP was the United Kingdom (8.3%). In four of the countries, 100% of the populace was insured; in Germany less than 1% was uninsured, and in the Netherlands less than 2%; in the United States, 16% of the populace was uninsured (rising to 25% of the populace if one considered those who at any time were uninsured). All countries except the United States had universal comprehensive minimum health benefits, and all but the United States and Canada had prescription drug benefits. With regard to primary care physicians, the dismal performance of the United States health-care system was apparent also. The percent of primary care practices that had a financial incentive for providing quality care was lowest in the United States (30%) and highest in the United Kingdom (95%). The percent of primary care practices using electronic medical records was also lowest in the United States and Canada (28 and 23%, respectively), while all other countries except Germany (42%) had electronic medical records in 79% to 98% of primary care practices.[75]

That the United States spends over 50% more on health care in terms of GDP, and over twice as much in terms of dollars, as any of the other six developed nations is well known. Perhaps nearly as well known is the fact that the United States is the only developed country without a comprehensive national minimum health benefit package and insurance coverage for the vast majority of its citizens (> 98%). Likely less appreciated are the findings that the United States ranks lowest in percent of primary care practices with a financial incentive for quality health-care delivery and use of electronic medical records (apart from Canada). Interestingly, Canada and Germany ranked nearly as poorly on these two measures as the United States; all three countries were the only ones not requiring patients to register with a primary care physician and seek a referral from their primary care physician before seeing a specialist (although Australia does not require registration with a primary care physician).

The conclusions of this extensive survey of the health-care experience of adults in seven developed countries are contained in the authors' abstract:

> In all countries, the study finds that having a "medical home" that is accessible and helps coordinate care is associated with significantly more positive experiences ... Patient-reported errors were high for those seeing multiple doctors or having multiple chronic illnesses. The United States stands out for cost-related access barriers and less-efficient care.[75]

The lesson across multiple developed countries with regard to effective health care seems clear: some form of the patient-centered medical home (PCMH) concept is important to maximize patient satisfaction while minimizing cost.

The lead article in the Fall/Winter 2008 issue of *AANS Neurosurgeon* (the publication of the American Association of Neurological Surgeons intended for neurosurgeons, not a public or research audience) was entitled "A Global Experience: Neurosurgeons Analyze Their Practice Environments."[76] The article considered health-care insurance and health-care costs in nine developed countries (Australia, Germany, Italy, Japan, South Korea, Sweden, Switzerland, the United Kingdom, and the United States) from a neurosurgical perspective. The United States was the only country with any uninsured citizens (over 15%). Health-care expenditures as a percent of GDP ranged from 8% (Japan) to 11% (Switzerland), with the outlier again being the United States at 16%. The mechanism for health-care insurance is largely or completely government-based in most countries: 100% in Australia, Sweden, and the United Kingdom (with alternative optional private insurance and limited co-payments by the patient) and 70–90% government-based in Germany, Italy, Japan, and South Korea (with the remainder being private insurance and/or patient co-payments). The United States had roughly 45% government-based health insurance and 35% private, with the remainder being out-of-pocket expenses for the individual (co-payments and uninsured charges to the patient). Switzerland was somewhat unique in having an individual mandate that requires each citizen to purchase health insurance from one of many (nearly one hundred) not-for-profit insurance companies. Insurance premiums vary based on whether a high-deductible or low-deductible plan is chosen (but not by age or preexisting conditions), and citizens with a low income can receive government support when the insurance premium exceeds roughly 10% of one's income. As in other countries, there are both public and private hospitals where one can choose to have treatment. Interestingly, the Swiss health-care system has perhaps the lowest amount of direct government involvement in health-care funding and delivery but combines universal coverage and relatively low overall cost with health-care outcomes that are among the best in the world.[76,77]

We saw similar data in the report cited earlier in this chapter considering adults' health-care experiences in seven countries. The immediate statistic is that the United States is the only one of the nine developed countries in Europe and Asia without universal health-care coverage. Second, the cost of health care in the United States is at least 50% greater than that of any of the other developed countries, despite the fact that by commonly accepted measures of effectiveness of health care (e.g., life expectancy and infant mortality), the United States ranks lower than many developing countries that spend far less on health care (e.g., Cuba):

	United States	Cuba
Life Expectancy at Birth (years/rank)[1]	78.3 / #36	78.3 / #36 (tie)
Infant Mortality (per 1,000 live births/rank)[2]	6.9 / #29	5.8 / #27
Total Health Expenditure (% of GDP/per capita)[3]	16.2 / $7,410	11.8 / $503

[1] United Nations (2005–2010) [2] US Centers for Disease Control (2004) [3] WHO (2009)

Physicians in the United States Contribute to the Disparity in Health Care

One can use these data as an indictment of the health-care delivery system in the United States—both from the aspect of expense and from the aspect of uninsured persons in the populace. However, the article immediately preceding the one cited earlier in this chapter in the same issue of *AANS Neurosurgeon* was entitled "Two Studies Show Economic Impact of Physician Practices: Physicians Generate Billions in Payroll and Millions in Taxes."[78] It reported data that "each private practice physician supported thirteen additional jobs, $640,000 in personal income for those jobs, and nearly $1.5 million in total economic activity." Moreover, "financial losses for treating Medicaid and uninsured patients were calculated at more than half a million dollars per physician."

The point of presenting these data is that in the United States, health care has become an economic rather than humanitarian enterprise—and that physicians have become engulfed in the "profiteering tsunami."

Do we maintain local police and fire departments in order to "generate billions in payroll and millions in taxes"?

Do we see data on the "economic losses" of educating children whose parents' incomes are too low for them to pay taxes?

I believe it is a sad commentary when professional medical journals need to justify each physician's activity in terms of economic benefit or attempt to create a sense of guilt in the populace as a whole for the large amount of "unreimbursed care" each physician provides.

Equally disturbing is the elitist view of the medical specialty boards in the United States. For example, the American Board of Neurological Surgery, which sets the examination standards and criteria for granting board certification to neurosurgeons licensed in the United States, refuses to recognize training received by neurosurgery residents (physicians-in-training to become a neurosurgeon) outside of North America. There are world-class neurosurgery training programs in many places throughout the world (Europe and Asia in particular) whose faculty, medical resources, and research productivity match any program in the United States. Despite this, a US neurosurgeon-in-training cannot take advantage of these excellent programs as part of their formal training in order to broaden both their neurosurgical education as well as their cultural awareness of what is happening in other countries.

The European Association of Neurosurgical Societies (EANS), with considerable effort and diplomacy, has established standards for neurosurgical training throughout the European Union (EU).[79] The EANS has established the European Examination in Neurosurgery, part I consisting of a written examination and part II an oral examination. This two-part examination structure is modeled in large part on the American Board of Neurological Surgery's (ABNS) two-part examination for determining that a neurosurgeon can be board certified. Like its United States counterpart, the European Examination in Neurosurgery does not give a neurosurgeon license to practice neurosurgery—but it does acknowledge that "the holder has achieved a good level in the theory and practice of neurosurgery." If the EANS and the ABNS could join forces regarding neurosurgical certification, it is likely that a worldwide certification standard for neurosurgery could be realized.

In Europe, many of the premier neurosurgical training programs are educating promising young neurosurgeons from around the world (not just from fellow EU countries). Each "foreign" neurosurgeon-in-training gains not only neurosurgical expertise but also gains cultural awareness of his or her host country during that period of training. In the United States, neurosurgeon-in-training visitors from foreign countries are limited to observation of surgical procedures (i.e., none of the "hands-on" neurosurgical training that is essential for the acquisition of surgical skills) or laboratory research. At least these guests from other countries, while training in the United States, can go out with their American colleagues and have a beer together! Otherwise, it would be simpler and cheaper to provide their neurosurgical experience from the United States solely via the Internet (videos, teleconferences, etc.).

Again, in the United States, are neurosurgeons in particular—and physicians in general—sensitive to the universal aspect of health care as implied by the Hippocratic Oath? Does the delivery of health care (in terms of training fellow physicians) stop at a country's border? We can communicate using the Internet, make phone calls, wire money, and travel by plane throughout the world. Why can't we have reputable physicians-in-training from around the world seek medical education at the most appropriate reputable institution—wherever that institution may be throughout the world—for each of them?

Perhaps it is time for "Doctors Without Borders" to be not only a worldwide humanitarian effort but a worldwide medical education effort as well.

Chapter 21: "Listen to the Doctor, Listen to the Patient"—Trends in Restoring the Doctor–Patient Relationship

We saw in chapter 7 that there has been a trend over the past two decades to use hospital-based physicians (hospitalists), who work on fixed shifts and typically sign off their ten to twenty (or more) patients every shift to another hospitalist physician. Hospitalists generally take over the care of patients from primary (office-based) physicians when the primary care physician's patients are admitted to the hospital. We also saw there are data being accumulated that one of the main motivations behind the hospitalist movement—saving money—may not in fact be the case; once the costs of patient care beyond the hospitalization are included, it is likely that hospitalists cost the health-care system more than having the hospitalized patient taken care of by his or her primary physician.

But another compelling issue with this arrangement is summarized by the quote in chapter 7 from a patient:

A good primary physician is a permanent part of your life. To hospitalists, if you drop dead on the way home, they've still done their job.[15]

Patients realize that continuity of care—having one physician who can say, "the buck stops here" (and who can be held personally accountable)—is important in the overall efficacy of health-care delivery. Perhaps patients need to be consulted more in the evaluation of health-care delivery in the United States.

I am frequently asked by patients who participate in (or who have family members who participate in) the Kaiser Permanente health-care system, "Can you help me get to see a Kaiser neurosurgeon?" The Kaiser system has significant advantages over US health-care delivery in general, such as the fact that the uniform information technology allows immediate access to a patient's medical records (including imaging such as CT, MRI, and ultrasound scans) by any physician in the Kaiser system. Additionally, the regionalization of specialist care should make for significant reductions in duplication of services and high-tech (high-expense) medical equipment. For example, in Northern California the Kaiser health-care system concentrates its neurosurgeons primarily in two hospitals, although there are twenty-four Kaiser and Kaiser-affiliated hospitals throughout Northern California.

For many physicians who choose to work in the Kaiser system, one of the attractive aspects is the fixed work schedule—the physician knows exactly when he or she will be "on duty." However, given that specialist care tends to be more expensive than primary care, there appears to be a tendency to avoid referral to a specialist unless the condition is perceived as extremely urgent by the primary physician. The specialist has no reason to see a patient outside of the fixed office hours; if the condition is perceived as truly urgent by the patient, that patient will show up in the emergency room. It would be informative to have accurate data on how often patient care is compromised because the fixed duty hours and salaried primary physician (or specialist, for that matter) delays evaluation and treatment in situations that are felt to be less than truly emergent. My impression over the years is that it is not infrequently that patients with serious but not life-and-death emergency conditions are not cared for as rapidly in a system (such as Kaiser) where the physicians—primary and specialist—are on fixed working schedules. In part, this suboptimal evaluation and treatment is likely due to the patient not being "a permanent part" of any physician's life.

In addition to considering the patient's opinion regarding the doctor–patient relationship, it might be helpful to examine the opinions of physicians-in-training regarding their own education. As an example, I here consider the regulation of duty hours for neurosurgeons-in-training (neurosurgical residents).

To review the various limitations on hours that a resident physician may work—both legislation and proposals—would comprise a lengthy chapter itself. However, in summary, to address the potential for medical errors made by residents who were exhausted because of overly long work hours, across-the-board limitations were proposed (and enacted in 2003) that a work shift must be limited to sixteen hours at a time, and total hours worked must be limited to eighty hours per week. Over the past decade, several committees have addressed this issue:

- Accreditation Council for Graduate Medical Education (ACGME) Work Group on Resident Duty Hours (2002)
- Institute of Medicine Committee on Optimizing Graduate Medical Trainee Hours and Work Schedules to Improve Patient Safety (2008)
- ACGME Task Force on Quality Care and Professionalism (2009)

In response to the restrictions on resident duty hours, a report approved by three major US neurosurgical organizations (Society of Neurological Surgeons, American Board of Neurological Surgery, and Residency Review Committee for Neurological Surgery) published in 2009 offered a number of comments.[12] They argued that the restrictions on resident duty hours (especially if additional restrictions were imposed) would detrimentally affect resident competence as well as continuity of care. The restrictions would also detrimentally affect the infrastructure of neurosurgical training programs by diluting the residents' education and experience (in part because "physician extenders," such as physician assistants and nurse practitioners, would need to be employed to assume patient care in the residents' absence). These additional personnel would result in significant additional costs to training programs as well. The primary goal of the report was to convince the ACGME and other involved parties that neurosurgery residency training required a balance between restricted duty hours in order to minimize errors resulting from fatigue and sufficient duty hours to allow for adequate resident education and mastery of the complex surgical and decision-making skills required for successful neurosurgery.

This serves as an introduction to a recent survey of neurosurgery residents' opinions regarding the duty hour restrictions they should be subjected to.[80] This survey was conducted by members of the Department of Neurosurgery (both faculty and residents), University of Florida, and consisted of a questionnaire sent to every neurosurgery training program director in the United States and Puerto Rico (101 programs), to be distributed to all the neurosurgery residents in each training program (approximately 1,100 residents in all). The response rate was 34% (377 residents), a reasonable figure for this type of survey. The eighteen questions included in the survey and the responses (in percentages) are given in tabular form in the article; the responses to most questions were in the form of five choices (strongly agree, agree, neutral, disagree, strongly disagree). In the discussion that follows, the results for strongly agree and agree and also for disagree and strongly disagree are combined for simplicity of comparison.

As an indicator, perhaps, of the particular dedication of neurosurgery residents to their specialty, nearly three out of four residents (74%) disagreed that neurosurgery residents should be subjected to the same duty hour restrictions as residents in other specialties, such as internal medicine; only 15% agreed. Regarding the further reduction in work hours proposed by the ACGME—all within the previously imposed eighty-hours-per-week work limit—from a maximum of thirty hours at a time (twenty-four unrestricted hours plus six hours for additional responsibilities but not work in patient clinics) to a maximum of twenty-eight hours (twenty-four hours plus four hours), the majority of neurosurgery residents disagreed that the reduction would lead either to a reduction in resident fatigue or to the prevention of medical errors (59% disagreed and 22% agreed regarding fatigue, 64% disagreed and 14% agreed regarding medical errors). With a further reduction in work hours, patient familiarity and continuity of care was felt to be adversely affected by 73% of residents and positively affected by only 4%. Regarding the effect of more patient sign-outs to another physician (or ancillary staff) on the increased likelihood of medical errors if resident work hours were reduced further, 63% felt errors would increase whereas only 4% felt such errors would decrease. Overall, 74% of neurosurgery residents felt that the proposed further reduction in work hours would have a negative impact on their training; only 8% felt the reduction would have a positive impact. However, the strongest disagreement with the proposed further reduction in work hours came with regard to "surgical opportunities and educational experiences"—fully 85% of neurosurgery residents felt the reduction would be detrimental, whereas less than 4% felt the reduction would be beneficial.[80]

There are also data indicating that the duty hour regulations have a negative effect on other measures of the neurosurgical educational experience (as detailed in chapter 7). The scores of neurosurgery residents taking the American Board of Neurological Surgery written examination declined significantly from 2002 (before the duty hour limitations were instituted) to 2006. Moreover, although the number of residents attending the annual meeting of the American Association of Neurological Surgeons increased from 2002 to 2007, the percentage of resident attendees making a presentation at the annual meeting (a measure of research productivity by residents) declined, also significantly, from 85% to 66%.[12]

One aspect of physician training that has not been addressed in detail is the effect of restricted duty hours on the physician (or surgeon) with regard to on-the-job professional competency after training. If the physician-in-training has less experience with late-night emergencies (surgical or otherwise), will that physician be as competent as a physician who dealt with such emergencies more frequently during the training years? One of the valuable lessons from the chairman of my neurosurgical training program was, "Deal with neurosurgical emergencies as a resident enough times when you are a bit tired or stressed, and you will likely do the right thing after residency when you are a bit tired or stressed and on your own." Unfortunately, one does not learn good medical/surgical habits while at home sleeping. This point has been emphasized by several senior neurosurgeons in an article cited in chapter 7:

> When a patient decides to undergo a complex procedure ... he/ she expects that the neurosurgeon will have the ability to see the procedure through to the end. The ability to do this does not develop overnight, but instead is the product of many years of training and psychomotor conditioning. The neurosurgeon-in-training learns over time what his or her limits are and develops the ability to patiently complete a microsurgical procedure where intense concentration and psychomotor persistence are required until the task is finished.[13]

A neurosurgery resident in particular (and in-training physicians in other specialties in their own different ways) must during his or her half-dozen or more years of training acquire not only the complex psychomotor skills necessary to complete a neurosurgical procedure that may last up to a dozen hours or more but also the ability to make rapid decisions upon which the life of another human being depends. Moreover, the resident must learn his or her own limitations in order to avoid situations detrimental to the patient. It is telling that the most vigorous opponents to the somewhat arbitrary and bureaucratic decisions regarding limitations on the duty hours for the training of physicians (neurosurgeons in particular) are the neurosurgery residents themselves—followed closely by the majority of their senior neurosurgery faculty mentors (who have clearly dedicated their lives to the care of patients and the education of residents).

Neurosurgery residents by a ratio of more than 20:1 indicated, as noted above, that the proposed further reduction in their work hours would negatively impact their "surgical opportunities and educational experiences." Physicians-in-training are salaried and not paid by the hour. This is one of the very few aspects of American medicine that appears to be driven not by the profit motive but rather by the desire of the resident to be the best physician one can be.

Postscript

The groups that brought about the conception and birth of the United States as a country in the late 1700s were the disenfranchised and the young. The same groups—the disenfranchised populace (with regard to health care) and the young (physicians-in-training)—are leading the charge for true health-care reform in the United States at present.

When the "Occupy Health Care Movement" takes hold, it is likely that patients (i.e., the health-care-consuming populace as a whole) and residents (physicians-in-training) will be at the forefront!

Epilogue: Health versus Wealth? Health = Wealth? Physician, Heal Thyself!

We began with the Hippocratic Oath, that pillar of Western medicine and the prospectus for what the doctor–patient relationship could be.

We saw how the training of physicians, rather than nurturing the doctor–patient relationship, has become the inoculation of the for-profit "virus" into the budding physician. The physician-in-training learns that personal financial success in medicine is tied to the financial success of drug companies and medical device manufacturers—not to the success of the physician's efforts to heal patients.

In oftentimes subtle ways, corporate America has virtually incorporated itself into the physician's professional "genome." Physicians are offered free samples and training courses that are thinly disguised vacations, and they are now expected to collect co-payments from their patients at each visit that often exceed the reimbursement to the physician from the patient's insurance company.

We learned that models of health-care delivery have been developed not to improve the doctor–patient relationship but rather to erode that relationship in the interests of the doctor's time schedule and quality of life. The data regarding the effectiveness of removing the "one patient–one physician" relationship in terms of saving health-care dollars in the long run are as of yet inconclusive at best. Clearly the doctor–patient relationship suffers when the patient's doctor morphs into a team of doctors that hand the patient from one doctor to another throughout a hospitalization—a team that often has limited interaction with the patient's primary physician.

Madison Avenue advertising of prescription drugs direct to consumers— never a cost-effective generic drug; always the most profitable, expensive new drug (with only a short-term track record on safety)—serves the corporate bottom line more than the consumer's health (both medical health and financial health). Medical device manufacturers have similarly used various tactics to enhance the utilization of expensive implantable devices, often at the expense of both the health-care dollar and the health-care consumer (i.e., the patient).

We saw how government policies often impede rather than facilitate truly cost-effective health care. Well-intended government regulations may backfire in practice (e.g., the EMTALA rules that hospitals learn to skirt around in the interests of their own cost saving) rather than improve either the cost saving of the entire health-care system or the welfare of the individual patient. Food and Drug Administration policies that limit the FDA's role to ensuring that drug and device company research is reasonably safe (even if unlikely to be efficacious) have allowed greedy companies to squander millions of research dollars on clinical trials that were doomed to fail. Through patents and acquisition of start-up companies with valuable intellectual property, large medical drug/device corporations have thwarted the rapid development of novel, more cost-effective and potentially life-saving drugs and devices in order to capitalize on their currently profitable drugs or devices, which still have years left under patent protection.

The plethora of new techniques and implants for various disorders of the lumbar spine have demonstrated the supremacy of the profit motive—for surgeons, hospitals, and medical device companies—over the patient's long-term health benefit. The burgeoning cost of health care for disorders of the lumbar spine is not the patient's fault, but rather it is the fault of those in the health-care system who fail to put the patient ahead of the profit. As in so many other areas of US medicine, the "crony capitalism" of for-profit entities involved in the treatment of disorders of the lumbar spine resembles the "crony capitalism" of the Wall Street–style financial system that created the recent mortgage meltdown and general financial crisis on both sides of the Atlantic. In both instances, the profits are privatized while the losses are socialized.

Physicians and physicians' professional organizations have themselves succumbed to the profit motive rather than maintaining commitment to the

Hippocratic Oath. Turf wars between physicians with competing surgical techniques have allowed personal financial gain to trump what is the best for the patient. Some medical professional organizations have reinvented themselves; no longer agents for furthering the medical education of their physician members, they have found a need to become the "educator" for their physician members on how to maximize the individual physician's financial success (rather than be the "educator" on how the individual physician can best treat his or her patients).

We looked at both health-care delivery and the training of physicians in other developed nations. The United States is the only such country without some form of universal health care. Until we in the United States acknowledge that health care is part of a civilized society (much like education, fire, and police protection), the costs of health care—and the quality of health care—in the United States will continue to diverge. Costs will increase while quality will decrease as the various parties involved (drug/device manufacturers, hospitals, physicians) each becomes more and more sophisticated at gaming the system—and each spends more and more resources on lobbying elected officials.

"Socialized medicine"—like the emperor's new clothes—is merely a ruse to frighten the populace into maintaining a for-profit health-care system that ultimately will bankrupt the United States financially, medically, and socially. At present we do indeed have "socialized medicine" in the United States, but unfortunately the socialized beneficiary is the for-profit health-care system at the expense of the citizen/patient!

We considered some interventions to reverse the present trend in the United States of health care becoming increasingly profit-centered rather than patient-centered. Returning health-care delivery to the local level (similar to local school districts)—rather than having all health care be determined by huge (often national) hospital chains, health-care insurers, and physicians' groups—can return the physician to the role of providing health care to individual patients over time instead of the physician being just another node in a massive health-care delivery network. The PCMH concept is a step in this direction, but critics claim that the cost of converting the health-care system in the United States to a PCMH model is too expensive (despite evidence to the contrary from other developed countries). Statewide, nationwide, and, indeed in the future, even international consortiums of individual hospitals and hospital groups and physicians and physician groups (medical organizations) can gather and, in turn, disseminate the latest data on "best practices" in topics ranging from preventive medicine to personalized medicine and genomics. The European Association for Predictive, Preventive, and Personalized Medicine (EPMA)—already worldwide in scope—is another step in the right direction.

Lastly, there are signs that patients (i.e., the general population) desire a patient-centered health-care delivery system and a strengthened patient–physician relationship (rather than a patient–financial intermediary–physician relationship). And in a prophetic return to the "youth" of medicine—where we started this consideration of health care in the United States—physicians-in-training are demanding such a return to the quintessential patient–physician relationship as well.

I will conclude with a lesson from a society on a small, previously remote Pacific island. (The term "remote" is scarcely applicable to any part of the planet in this age of both worldwide travel—of people and of viruses—and the universal effects of global warming.) For millennia, the inability of an island-dwelling person to escape one's homeland—sometimes an atoll measured in square meters rather than square kilometers—forced the inhabitants of these islands to become very savvy at interpersonal relations. The option of escape (or banishment, e.g., "outside the Roman Empire") did not exist, and the option of mortal revenge or "genocide" in a population numbering in the hundreds (or even dozens) made the prospect of one's own survival after exterminating one's enemies quite remote. The politicians from these sea-locked specks in the Pacific were the most polished I have seen with respect to interpersonal relations. If a *faux pas* destroyed one's political career, there was no option of becoming a TV political commentator, joining a prominent law firm, or becoming a Washington, DC, lobbyist.

<u>The year: 1967.</u> The Vietnam War (which the Vietnamese now—more appropriately—refer to as the "American War") was at its height.

<u>The place: Palau.</u> The Palau Island group is located about 800 km east of the southern Philippine island of Mindanao, 2,400 km east of southern Vietnam, and 3,200 km south of Tokyo. Presently an independent nation (since 1994, the Republic of Palau), Palau was in 1967 part of the United Nations' Trust Territory of the Pacific Islands, administered by the United States.

<u>The venue: An evening in a Palauan village.</u> Shortly after I arrived in Palau as a Peace Corps Volunteer, one evening some of the males in the village—ranging from preteens to village elders—gathered to play "hanafuda." Hanafuda ("flower cards" in Japanese) is a card game that was the equivalent of poker in the late nineteenth century for the Yakuza (the Japanese Mafia). Later, hanafuda lost its underworld connotations, and presently hanafuda—under various names and various formats—is enjoyed as a card game in many countries throughout the Asia-Pacific region.

At the start of the game in the Palauan village, each player received a pile of matchsticks—the equivalent of poker chips. Hanafuda is a game of chance as much as of skill, and so a novitiate like me could look reasonably facile just by memorizing the names of the cards and the winning combinations. As we played the game through the evening (with the requisite conversation and beers—San Miguel from the Philippines and Kirin from Japan), naturally some players lost matchsticks and others won. Whenever one player had lost all his "chips," the player with the most "chips," rather than being declared the winner, would redistribute his "winnings" among those with the fewest matchsticks (including the "matchless" loser). No matter whom the winner was—the village chief or the village dolt, the eldest or the youngest—the matchsticks were always redistributed equally. The object was not to win, but rather to enjoy the game—to have a forum for enjoyable interaction and conversation for everyone. If one individual were to claim victory (not that a large pile of matchsticks was much of a prize!), not only would the game be over, but (more importantly) it would replace the camaraderie of the mutually enjoyed experience with the bitterness of game-ending competition. Of course each person enjoyed "winning" (there was no shortage of excitement, cheering, and moaning), but the paramount goal was that "the game must go on."

Perhaps the Palauan version of hanafuda was more like the modern day Olympics—repeated every four years for all nations—than the gladiator contests to the death that characterized the Roman coliseums. No doubt there is a lesson to be learned as one, sitting in the ruins of a Roman coliseum, ponders the finite nature of "mortal combat for sport."

There is a lesson in this for the present-day physician in America: Look not upon your patient as the source of your income (through the patient's insurance and co-payments), so long as you provide medical service according to the "latest American Medical Association guidelines." In the long run, medical care is not about "winning" personally in a financial sense; it is about the patient's quality of life. Your long-term success as a physician will depend on your doctor–patient relationships—established, nurtured, and maintained one patient at a time. The Palauans knew that enjoying the game—keeping everyone part of the competition over time— was more important than any one person winning in the short run. This is crucial to the "healing art and science of medicine." If the physician's financial gain (or that of the hospital, the drug or device company, or the health insurance company) stands in the way of minimizing the patient's suffering, the long-term consequences are devastating. Just as families (and ethnic groups) remember the unjustified death of a relative at the hands of a ruthless dictator (or, on a larger scale, ethnic genocide), financial gains of the health-care industry that are made at the expense of the patient's health (individually and collectively in the population as a whole) are not forgotten.

One could argue that the doctor–patient relationship is the most intimate relationship possible between two people. Certainly this is true in neurosurgery, where the surgeon holds not only the person's life in his or her hands, but perhaps more importantly, the person's quality of life as well (i.e., whether that person will be as functionally intact—physically and mentally—as possible.) To allow personal economic benefit to enter into this relationship—as has been demonstrated throughout this book—is equivalent to medical prostitution.

To date, physicians as a group have not been vigorous defendants of the lofty goals of the Hippocratic Oath that we all have sworn to. Until each of us, as individual physicians and as members of professional medical societies, takes the bold step to renounce the techniques of for-profit medicine that have infected American medicine over the past fifty years, the "joy of healing those who seek my help" will increasingly elude physicians:

— Provide the treatment that is best for the patient—not what is best financially for the physician.
— Provide the same care to every patient that one would provide to a close family member.
— Reject rather than embrace the corrupt techniques that have consumed the political process in America (e.g., the medical lobbyists in state capitals and in Washington, DC).
— Reject industry offers, whether they be free educational courses that are disguised vacations, support for research of questionable benefit, or offers to participate in trials where the goal is clearly to demonstrate a statistical (and financial) benefit rather than a medical benefit.
— Educate patients and elected officials alike as to the areas throughout the health-care delivery system where profit has trumped the care of the patient.
— Embrace, not hinder, valid progress in health-care delivery.

Health-care reform should start—not end—with physicians. Let the healing begin!

Bibliography

1. Kuhn TS. *The Structure of Scientific Revolutions*. Chicago: The University of Chicago Press, 1996.

2. Reich R. *Supercapitalism*. New York: Vintage, 2007, 224.

3. "Hippocratic Oath: Modern Version." Accessed 10/13/12 via the National Library of Medicine, National Institutes of Health website to the Public Broadcasting Service website. Last modified 03/27/01. http://www.pbs.org/wgbh/nova/body/hippocratic-oath-today.html.

4. Martin WF. Long HW, Culbertson RA, Beyt E. "The Master of Medical Management (MMM) degree: an analysis of alumni perceptions." J Health Admin Educ 24 (2007): 391–398.

5. "Master of Medical Management Program Overview." Accessed 10/13/12 at the University of Southern California Marshall School of Business website. http://www.marshall.usc.edu/mmm.

6. Hiraoka K, Meguro K, Mori E. "Prevalence of idiopathic normal pressure hydrocephalus in the elderly population of a Japanese rural community." Neuro Med Chir 48 (2008): 197–200.

7. Sullivan SE, Benzil DL. "A treatable dementia: what neurosurgeons should know about NPH." AANS Neurosurgeon 19 #1 (2010): 16–17.

8. Stein SC, Burnett MG, Sonnad SS. "Shunts in normal pressure hydrocephalus: do we place too many or too few?" J Neurosurg 105 (2006): 815–822.

9. Medicare Part B 2012 fee schedules for Santa Clara County (Silicon Valley), California. Accessed 11/19/12 at the Medicare reimbursement website. http://www.palmettoGBA.com.

10. Hatlen TJ, Shurtleff DB, Loeser JD, Ojemann JG, Avellino AM, Ellenbogen RG. "Nonprogrammable and programmable cerebrospinal fluid shunt valves: a 5-year study." J Neurosurg Pediatrics 9 (2012): 462–467.

11. Williams D. "Free drug data for doctors comes at a price." *San Jose Mercury News*, July 31, 2011.

12. Jagannathan J, Vates GE, Pouratian N, Sheehan JP, Patrie J, Grady MS, Jane Sr. JJ. "Impact of the Accreditation Council for Graduate Medical Education work-hour regulations on neurosurgical resident education and productivity." J Neurosurg 110 (2009): 820–827.

13. Dumont TM, Rughani AI, Penar PL, Horgan MA, Tranmer BI, Jewell RP. "Increased rate of complications on a neurological surgery service after implementation of the Accreditation Council for Graduate Medical Education work-hour restriction." J Neurosurg 116 (2012): 483–486.

14. Grady MS, Batjer HH, Dacey RG. "Resident duty hour regulation and patient safety: establishing a balance between concerns about resident fatigue and adequate training in neurosurgery." J Neurosurg 110 (2009): 828–836.

15. Span P. "Do hospitalists save money?" *New York Times*, August 12, 2011.

16. Kuo Y-F, Goodwin JS. "Association of hospitalist care with medical utilization after discharge: evidence of cost shift from a cohort study." Ann Intern Med 115 (2011): 152–159.

17. Roberts PA, Pollay M, Engles C, Pendleton B, Reynolds E, Stevens FA. "Effect on intracranial pressure of furosemide combined with varying doses and administration rates of mannitol." J Neurosurg 66 (1987): 440–446.

18. Andrews RJ, Rivera JO. "Optimizing mannitol and furosemide in the treatment of increased intracranial pressure." Congress of Neurological Surgeons 51st Annual Meeting, 2011.

19. Coronado VG, Xu L, Basavaraju SV, McGuire LC, Wald MM, Faul MD, Guzman BR, Hemphill JD. "Surveillance for traumatic brain injury-related deaths—United States, 1997–2007." Centers for Disease Control and Prevention Morbidity and Mortality Weekly Report 60 No 5 (2011): 1–32.

20. Roger VL, Go AS, Lloyd-James DM, Adams RJ, Berry JD, Brown TM, et al. "Heart disease and stroke statistics—2011 update." Circulation 123 (2011): e18–e209.

21. Schoepp DD. "Where will new neuroscience therapies come from?" Nature Reviews Drug Discovery 10 (2011): 715–716.

22. Weinstein JN, Lurie JD, Olson P, Bronner KK, Fisher ES, Morgan TS. "United States trends and regional variations in lumbar spine surgery: 1992–2003." Spine 31 (2006): 2707–2714.

23. Deyo RA, Mirza SK, Martin BI, Kreuter W, Goodman DC, Jarvik JG. "Trends, major medical complications, and charges associated with surgery for lumbar stenosis in older adults." J Am Med Assoc 303 (2010): 1259–1265.

24. Burton CV. "The history of lumbar spine stabilization (usually referred to as 'fusion')." Accessed 10/13/12 at The Burton Report website. http://www.burtonreport.com.

25. Deyo RA, Gray DT, Kreuter W, Mirza S, Martin BI. "United States trends in lumbar fusion surgery for degenerative conditions." Spine 30 (2005): 1441–1445.

26. Cheng JS, Lee MJ, Massicotte E, Ashman B, Gruenberg M, Pilcher LE, Skelly AC. "Clinical guidelines and payer policies on fusion for the treatment of chronic low back pain." Spine 36 (2011): S144–S163.

27. Babu MA, Coumans JV, Carter BS, Taylor WR, Kasper EM, Roitberg BZ, Krauss WE, Chen CC. "A review of lumbar spinal instrumentation: evidence and controversy." J Neurol Neurosurg Psychiatry 82 (2011): 948–951.

28. Weinstein JN, Forman JL, et al. "Surgical versus nonoperative treatment for lumbar disc herniation: four-year results for the spine patient outcomes research trial (SPORT)." Spine 33 (2008): 2789–2800.

29. Tosteson ANA, Skinner JS, Tosteson TD, Lurie JD, Andersson G, Berven S, Grove MR, Hanscom B, Wienstein JN. "The cost-effectiveness of surgical versus nonoperative treatment for lumbar disc herniation over two years: evidence from the spine outcomes research trial (SPORT)." Spine 33 (2008): 2108–2115.

30. Mayer HM, Brock M. "Percutaneous endoscopic discectomy: surgical technique and preliminary results compared to microsurgical discectomy." J Neurosurg 78 (1993): 216–225.

31. Wang B, Lü G, Patel AA, Ren P, Cheng I. "An evaluation of the learning curve for a complex surgical technique: the full endoscopic interlaminar approach for lumber disc herniations." Spine J 11 (2011): 122–130.

32. METRx™ Microdiscectomy System Fact Sheet. Accessed 10/13/12 at the Medtronic, Minneapolis, MN 55432 USA website. http://www .medtronic.com.

33. "What is endoscopic discectomy?" Accessed 10/13/12 from the Beth Israel Deaconess Medical Center, Boston, MA 02215 USA website. http://www.bidmc.org.

34. Casal-Moro R, Castro-Menéndez M, Hernández-Blanco M, Bravo-Ricoy JA, Jorge-Barreiro FJ. "Long-term outcome after microendoscopic diskectomy for lumbar disk herniation: a prospective clinical study with a 5-year follow-up." Neurosurgery 68 (2011): 1568–1575.

35. van den Akker ME, Arts MP, van den Hout WB, Brand R, Koes BW, Peul WC. "Tubular diskectomy vs. conventional microdiskectomy for the treatment of lumbar disk-related sciatica: cost utility analysis alongside a double-blind randomized controlled trial." Neurosurgery 68 (2011): 829–836.

36. Anekstein Y, Smorgick Y, Lotan R, Agar G, Shalmon E, Floman Y, Mirovsky Y. "Diabetes mellitus as a risk factor for the development of lumbar spinal stenosis." Israel Med Assoc J 12 (2010): 16–20.

37. Sénégas J, Vital J-M, Pointillart V, Mangione P. "Long-term actuarial survivorship analysis of an interspinous stabilization system." Eur Spine J 16 (2007): 1279–1287.

38. Hsu KY, Zucherman JF, Hartjen CA, Mehalic TF, Implicito DA, Martin MJ, et al. "Quality of life of lumbar stenosis-treated patients in whom the X-STOP interspinous device was implanted." J Neurosurg Spine 5 (2006): 500–507.

39. X-Stop Spacer. Accessed 10/13/12 at the Medtronic, Minneapolis, MN 55432 USA website. http://www.medtronic.com.

40. Skidmore G, Ackerman SJ, Bergin C, Ross D, Butler J, Suthar M, Rittenberg J. "Cost-effectiveness of the X-STOP interspinous spacer for lumbar spinal stenosis." Spine 36 (2011): E345–E356.

41. Sobottke R, Röllinghoff M, Siewe J, Schlegel U, Yagdiran A, Spangenberg M, et al. "Clinical outcomes and quality of life after open microsurgical decompression or implantation of an interspinous stand-alone space." Minim Invas Neurosurg 53 (2010): 179–183.

42. Tuschel A, Chavanne A, Eder C, Meissl M, Becker P, Ogon M. "Implant survival analysis and failure modes of the X-STOP interspinous distraction device." Spine epub Feb 2, 2011.

43. Epstein G. "Economic beat: still more on Fannie Mae and Freddie Mac." Barron's Jan 16, 2012: 49.

44. US Department of Health and Human Services (HHS), Centers for Medicare and Medicaid Services (CMS), Publication CMS-1063-F (2002): 11–12. Accessed on 10/13/12 at the CMS website. http://www.cms.gov.

45. US Department of Health and Human Services (HHS), Centers for Medicare and Medicaid Services (CMS), Publication CMS-1063-F (2002): 34–35. Accessed on 10/13/12 at the CMS website. http://www.cms.gov.

46. US Department of Health and Human Services (HHS), Centers for Medicare and Medicaid Services (CMS), Publication CMS-1063-F (2002): 238–239. Accessed on 10/13/12 at the CMS website. http://www.cms.gov.

47. Babu MA, Nahed BV, DeMoya MA, Curry WT. "Is trauma transfer influenced by factors other than medical need? An examination of insurance status and transfer in patients with mild head injury." Neurosurgery 69 (2011): 659–667.

48. American Medical Association Mission and Core Values. Accessed 10/13/12 at the American Medical Association website. https://www.ama-assn.org.

49. California Medical Association Mission Statement. Accessed 10/13/12 at the California Medical Association website. http://www.cmanet.org.

50. American College of Surgeons Mission Statement. Accessed 10/13/12 at the American College of Surgeons website. http://www.facs.org.

51. California Association of Neurological Surgeons Purpose. Accessed 10/13/12 at the California Association of Neurological Surgeons website. http://www.cans1.org.

52. American Medical Association About AMPAC. Accessed 10/13/12 at the American Medical Association website. https://www.ama-assn.org.

53. California Medical Association Political Action Committee (CALPAC). Accessed 10/13/12 at the California Medical Association website. http://www.cmanet.org.

54. The California Association of Neurological Surgeons Annual Meeting Programs for 1996 and 2011 are reproduced with permission from the California Association of Neurological Surgeons.

55. US Department of Labor Continuation of Health Coverage— COBRA. Accessed 10/13/12 at the US Department of Labor website. http://www.dol.gov.

56. National Resident Matching Program—Main Residency Match. Accessed 10/13/12 at the National Resident Matching Program website. http://www.nrmp.org.

57. *Mosby's Medical Dictionary*, 8th Edition. Philadelphia: Elsevier, 2009.

58. Hirsh L. "Corralling Costs." *Press-Enterprise*, Riverside, CA, Oct 1, 2009.

59. Healy WL. "Gainsharing: a primer for orthopaedic surgeons." J Bone Joint Surg Am 88 (2006): 1880–1887.

60. World Federation of Neurosurgical Societies Member Societies. Accessed 10/13/12 at the World Federation of Neurosurgical Societies website. http://www.wfns.org.

61. Steinmetz MP. "Significant threat ... Rapid response." Congress Quarterly 12 #4 (2011): 23.

62. Norwood E. "ERN/NCRA Vision." Accessed 10/13/12 at the Ed Norwood's LinkedIn website. http://www.linkedin.com.

63. MICRA - History. Accessed 10/13/12 at The Doctors Company website. http://www.thedoctorscompany.com.

64. CMA - MICRA. Accessed 10/13/12 at the California Medical Association website. http://www.cmanet.org.

65. Welcome to 23andMe. Accessed 1/10/12 at the 23andMe Inc. website. https://www.23andme.com.

66. Harrison C. "23andMe patent creates a stir." Nature Reviews Drug Discovery 11 (2012). 510–512.

67. Golubnitschaja O, Costigliola V. "European strategies in predictive, preventive and personalised medicine: highlights of the EPMA World Congress 2011." Accessed 1/10/12 at the EPMA website. http://www.epmanet.eu.

68. Golubnitschaja O, Costigliola V. "General report and recommendations in predictive, preventive and personalised medicine 2012: white paper

of the European Association of Predictive, Preventive and Personalised Medicine." Accessed 9/10/12 at the EPMA website. http://www .epmanet.eu.

69. Bitton A, Martin C, Landon BE. "A nationwide survey of patient-centered medical home demonstration projects." J Gen Intern Med 25 (2010): 584–592.

70. "Joint principles of the patient-centered medical home - February 2007." Accessed 10/13/12 at the Patient-Centered Primary Care Collaborative website. http://www.pcpcc.net.

71. "Standards and guidelines for NCQA's patient-centered medical home (PCMH) 2011." Accessed 10/13/12 at the National Committee for Quality Assurance website. http://www.ncqa.org.

72. "NCQA PCMH 2011 Brochure." Accessed 10/13/12 at the National Committee for Quality Assurance website. http://www.ncqa.org.

73. Rosenthal TC. "The medical home: growing evidence to support a new approach to primary care." J Am Board Fam Med 21 (2008): 427–440.

74. Nutting PA, Miller WL, Crabtree BF, Jaen CR, Stewart EE, Stange KC. "Initial lessons from the first national demonstration project on practice transformation to a patient-centered medical home." Ann Fam Med 7 (2009): 254–260.

75. Schoen C, Osborn R, Doty MM, Bishop M, Peugh J, Murukutla N. "Toward higher-performance health systems: adults' health care experiences in seven countries, 2007." Health Affairs 26 (2007): w717–w734.

76. Couldwell WT, Seaver MJ, Kaye A, Kawase T, Bertalanffy H, Koechlin N, Westphal M, Mathiesen T, Powell M. "A global experience: neurosurgeons analyze their practice environments." AANS Neurosurgeon 17 #3 (2008): 5–19.

77. "Healthcare in Switzerland." Accessed 10/13/12 at the Wikipedia website. http://en.wikipedia.org.

78. "Two studies show economic impact of physician practices: physicians generate billions in payroll and millions in taxes." AANS Neurosurgeon 17 #3 (2008): 3–4.

79. "European Association of Neurosurgical Societies / European Union of Medical Specialties Examination in Neurosurgery." Accessed 10/13/12 at the European Association of Neurosurgical Societies website. http://www.eans.org.

80. Fargen KM, Chakraborty A, Friedman WA. "Results of a National Neurosurgery Resident survey on duty hour regulations." Neurosurgery 69 (2011): 1162–1170.

Index

American Osteopathic Association
(AOA), 128
AMPAC (American Medical
Association Political Action
Committee), 100–101
AOA (American Osteopathic
Association), 128
Annals of Internal Medicine, 38
annual meetings, of professional
societies
  CANS 1996, 102–104
  CANS 2011, 105–108
  as focused on improving
    financial health of provider
    rather than health of patient,
    107
  overview, 101–102
Apollo Hospitals Group, 112
Apollo Telemedicine Networking
Foundation (ATNF), 112
ATNF (Apollo Telemedicine
Networking Foundation), 112
Australia, health care in, 132–135

B
Barron's, 78
Boerhringer-Ingelheim, 129
Bonner, John, 104
Borry, Pascal, 123
Bracco Group, 125
brain, decade of, 59–60
brain aneurysms, 89–92
brain tumors, 91–93

C
California
  hospital-based health care in, 43
  medical malpractice claims, 119

California Association of
Neurological Surgeons (CANS),
100, 102–107, 108
California Medical Association
(CMA), 99, 100, 119–120
California Medical Association
Political Action Committee
(CALPAC), 101
California Supreme Court, 120–121
The California Endowment, 129
CALPAC (California Medical
Association Political Action
Committee), 101
Canada, health care in, 132–134
CANS (California Association of
Neurological Surgeons), 100,
102–107, 108
cardiac pacemakers, 94
cardiologist, versus cardiac surgeon,
97
Carlson, Angela, 108
Carter, Bob, 106
CBF (cerebral blood flow), 52–54
Centers for Medicare and Medicaid
Services (CMS), 80
cerebral blood flow (CBF), 52–54
certification
  of continuing medical education,
    17
  in neurosurgery, 137
Charité Medical University, 124
Chestnut, Randall M., 104
Children's Health Insurance
Program (CHIP), 78
CHIP (Children's Health Insurance
Program), 78cigarettes, paradigm
shift in mass media advertising,
50–51
Cisco Systems, 112
Cleveland Clinic Foundation, 122

CPSIA information can be obtained at www.ICGtesting.com
Printed in the USA
LVOW132312090413

328431LV00003B/180/P